Preface

The tragedy of the HIV pandemic conceals many ironies. Foremost among these is that for so long the morbid social fascination with AIDS has gone hand-in-hand with conspicuous social denial. For years now we have had certain knowledge of how to prevent further needless HIV infections, yet while thousands continue to live and die with HIV infection and disease, the wider dissemination of such knowledge has met an invisible barrier of avoidance or, perhaps worse, apathy in the larger community. Another irony concerns the counselling of people with HIV. Too often those with HIV are construed as being extraordinary in vocabulary, thought and deed, somehow set apart from the rest of society by the circumstances of their exposure to this unseen enemy. It is true that social marginalizing has frequently complicated access to, and the ability to respond of those who have HIV, but the essential point is that people with HIV infection and disease are just as much a part of society as those without. This is why counsellors have such a crucial role in HIV management. Counsellors frequently form a critical 'bridging group' between patients and their own society, and between understanding about HIV transmission and behavioural change. Perhaps it is precisely because of this task that HIV counsellors have had a disparate membership of health advisers, psychologists, nurses, social workers, doctors, counsellors from other fields, and volunteers from all walks of life and interest. Documented HIV counselling has involved face-to-face contact with individuals, pairs, families and groups, and individual contact by telephone helplines. Counselling is also arguably provided by leaflets, posters, radio and television, and videos. Although these endeavours have a united aim - of informing about HIV, about avoiding its spread and providing support in view of its consequences - what has been lacking overall is clear guidance on demonstrably effective methods of exercising counselling interventions in different settings. While the content of much counselling is understood, the process of counselling has been neglected. This new book is thus a most welcome arrival. It presents a format and philosophy for counselling interventions with refreshing clarity and organization and the reader will find valuable and challenging lessons in every chapter. The case studies in particular illustrate the truism that in most practical respects HIV is a social phenomenon, the management of which cannot be divorced from the responses of the patient's society. Indeed, the depth of the authors' recorded experiences suggests that the lessons our patients so generously provide can and should meaningfully enrich the perspectives and methods of professionals for the sake of all who follow.

David Miller
University College and Middlesex School of Medicine

London 1988

Acknowledgements

We gratefully acknowledge the guidance and support of a number of colleagues over many years. Foremost is Dr Eleanor Goldman, Associate Specialist of the Royal Free Hospital Haemophilia Centre, who helped to develop and apply many of the ideas described in this book. Dr Peter Kernoff, Director of the Katherine Dormandy Haemophilia Centre and Haemostasis Unit, and his staff, who were initially sceptical colleagues, challenged and influenced our thinking. To them we are indebted for allowing these ideas to be tested. Dr Kernoff has been the impetus behind the book in that he has, for many years, encouraged us to put the ideas in writing.

We are privileged to be able to thank all levels of management of the Hampstead Health Authority who have given us time and resources to put the ideas into practice in the District AIDS Counselling Unit.

The time and painstaking work of those people who read early drafts of the book and helped us with their comments is very much appreciated. We would like to thank especially Dr Greta Forster, Dr Patricia Hewitt and Dr Caroline Lindsey. Many ideas described did not develop in isolation and we acknowledge the skill, expertise and guidance of Dr Elizabeth Miller, David Miller and Dr Anthony Pinching.

A special mention goes to Lucy Perry of the Hampstead Health Authority AIDS Counselling Unit and Elizabeth Boyd of the Royal Free Hospital Haemophilia Centre, who gave us every support during the writing of this book.

Our publisher, Brian Parker, of Science Press, and his colleagues Alison Eden and Monique Maxwell were enthusiastic about the project from the start. They provided motivation, resources and guidance. Monica Chard deciphered endless scripts with great efficiency.

Perhaps the greatest acknowledgement must go to the many patients, their partners and families who have shared with us their personal concerns and experiences. Many of these have been painful. We have also shared many lighter moments with our patients. At all times their reactions to these concerns and experiences have been inspiring and challenging and have taught us to continually review our ideas.

AIDS
A Guide to Clinical Counselling

Riva Miller

*AIDS Counselling Co-ordinator,
Hampstead Health Authority.
Senior Social Worker and Family Therapist,
Haemophilia Centre and Haemostasis Unit,
Royal Free Hospital,
London*

Robert Bor

*District AIDS Counsellor, Senior Clinical
Psychologist and Family Therapist.
Royal Free Hospital and School of Medicine,
Hampstead Health Authority,
London*

science press

British Library Cataloguing in Publication Data:
Miller, Riva
AIDS: a guide to clinical counselling
1. AIDS patients. Counselling
I Title   II Bor, Robert
362. I'9697
ISBN 1-870026-40-3

Editor: Monique Maxwell
Design: Mehmet Hussein/Medilink Design

Printed in the United Kingdom by Latimer Trend Company Limited, Plymouth, UK

When patients are referred to in the singular, 'he' rather than 'she' or 'he/she' is used. This
does not reflect any bias on the part of the authors or publisher but is merely a convenient
pronoun.

Contents

1
Introduction

Patients with AIDS/HIV will confront difficulties about themselves, their illness and their relationships. The aim of this book is to help health care professionals to think about and deal with the wide range of problems in a practical way. This, in turn, helps these patients to live with their condition and manage their relationships and circumstances.

The ideas and approaches outlined in this book are based on the experience of counselling in a clinical setting. AIDS is an illness, and in spite of its social, psychological and legal aspects, counselling is inextricably linked to medical care.

If some of the most dreaded issues related to HIV antibody testing, AIDS diagnosis, treatment, and even death, are addressed at an early and appropriate time, patients, families, and members of the health care team may be better prepared to deal with the problems they may face.

Counselling is important in AIDS/HIV infection because:

- There is no cure
- AIDS is almost always fatal
- HIV is infectious
- Those most at risk are the young
- There are fears arising from uncertainty and incomplete knowledge
- There is sometimes conflicting information
- Some co-ordination of care is needed because of the many different medical specialities involved in treatment
- Good patient management can prevent problems.

The term 'counsellor' is used here to refer to any health care professional engaged in talking to patients with AIDS/HIV, on a full- or part-time basis. This includes doctors, nurses, social workers, psychologists, physiotherapists and occupational therapists.

There are many ways of counselling, and each depends on the background of the professional and the nature of the problem. In this book, we have highlighted the particular relationship problems that exist for patients with AIDS/HIV infection and their families, lovers, colleagues and the health care team. These problems are closely associated with the social stigma attached to AIDS/HIV infection as well as being related to concerns about sexuality, confidentiality and clinical treatment.

This book will help the reader to:

- Understand the impact of AIDS/HIV on individuals at all stages of illness
- Consider what skills are necessary to address the many psychosocial aspects of the illness
- Take into account the relationship difficulties that may arise from an illness that is primarily transmitted through sexual activities
- Use a method of counselling based on a continuous reassessment of the changing circumstances of the patient
- Deal with various practical and political issues which may influence both counselling and the establishment of a counselling service.

The ideas contained in this book have to be assessed against a background of developing knowledge of AIDS/HIV infection as this has a bearing on the counselling task. The problems and concerns of patients may change if, for example, there were to be less social stigma attached to AIDS in the future. Despite the huge emotional and personal cost of AIDS there are some gains that are becoming apparent: standards of hygiene and nursing are being upgraded; personal resources and technical skills are enhancing other fields of patient care; and much is being learnt about human sexuality and relationships.

2
Background to clinical AIDS/ HIV counselling

A review of the following questions is fundamental to considering counselling in AIDS/HIV infection:

- What is counselling?
- Why counsel?
- Who should counsel?
- Who should be counselled?
- When to counsel?
- Where to counsel?

What is Counselling?

'Counselling' lends itself to many interpretations and can be seen as either a helping relationship or a set of structured activities. Central to the counselling process are some specific goals - for example, attaining an empathic understanding of the patient's problems, although this alone is not enough to help patients to cope.

There are various 'schools' of counselling (eg, psychoanalytic or behavioural) to which a counsellor might adhere and this would be reflected in the way the counselling is conducted. There is no clear delineation between counselling and psychotherapy and the main difference seems to be that psychotherapy focuses on psychological health and stability whereas counselling is pragmatic and diverse and is found in education, marriage guidance, pastoral services, personnel and hospitals, among many other settings.

The Department of Health and Social Security has issued guidelines stressing the importance of counselling in relation to testing for the HIV antibody. This test is now available in genitourinary medicine clinics, antenatal clinics and, increasingly, in the surgeries of general practitioners. HIV testing is also carried out in a growing number of hospital departments such as intensive care units, surgical units and labour wards. Irrespective of where testing is performed, counselling can help patients adjust to their condition, prepare them for bad news, educate them about how HIV is spread, and contribute to the co-ordination of medical and social care. The AIDS counsellor is often the translator between patients, lovers, family members and the health care team. It is in these conversations that problems are identified and consideration is given as to how best to deal with them.

Why Counsel in AIDS/HIV Infection?

AIDS is a life-threatening illness and the issues involved in AIDS/HIV infection may be painful, frightening and threatening to patients and health care staff. Counselling is needed because:

There is no cure Patients with AIDS/HIV infection may need opportunities to talk about how to live with a life-threatening illness and how to face death.

AIDS is almost always fatal Patients, their lovers and families have to cope with and adjust to chronic and, at times, acute and terminal illness. The adjustments are both practical and psychological and range from housing and financial issues, to views on treatment and resuscitation.

HIV is infectious It is likely that people infected with the virus will remain infected and infectious for life. In the absence of a cure, information about prevention and transmission is a very important part of counselling and patients must be made aware of the importance of not acquiring new infections, such as other sexually transmitted diseases.

Those most at risk are young Health and longevity have been assumed to belong to the young who, until recently, have not been the focus of major health concern. Effective ways of talking and listening to young people have to be found and this presents a challenge particularly to those not accustomed to addressing issues of sex and sexuality. A diagnosis of HIV may mean a loss of independence physically, psychologically and socially.

There are fears arising from uncertainty and incomplete knowledge Fears about AIDS/HIV infection may be both reasonable and unreasonable. There is, for example, the fact that an HIV antibody positive person can remain asymptomatic for many years and there is uncertainty about whether all those who are HIV antibody positive will inevitably develop AIDS.

There is conflicting information Patients may have different sources of the rapidly evolving information about AIDS/HIV infection. Counselling can help patients make sense of and manage the conflicting views they encounter.

Good management can contain problems If difficulties are identified early, it is possible to make plans with patients ahead of a crisis and make referrals, as appropriate, to other agencies and professionals. This can lead to more efficient use of time and resources. By offering prompt and adequate support, some psychiatric episodes may even be avoided.

Co-ordination is neeeded AIDS/HIV infection affects many parts of the body and several specialist medical teams may be treating the patient. This can cause management problems and confusion for the patient unless care is properly co-ordinated.

Who should Counsel?
Counselling in AIDS/HIV infection can be either a full-time commitment or form part of the caring role of health care professionals. These include:

In hospitals:

Doctors
Nurses

Health advisors in genitourinary medicine clinics
Medical and nursing staff in Occupational Health Units
Physiotherapists
Occupational therapists
Social workers
Psychotherapists
Family therapists
Psychologists
Hospital chaplains

Others who come across patients with AIDS/HIV in the course of their work and who may need some additional skills in talking and listening include:

Phlebotomists
Radiographers
Telephonists
Porters
Receptionists
Domestic staff

In the community:
General practitioners
District nurses
Community psychiatric nurses
Health visitors
Social workers
Dental practitioners
Oral hygienists
Family planning doctors and nurses
Environmental health officers
School doctors
Staff in voluntary agencies
Psychotherapists
Psychologists
Family therapists
Speech therapists

In blood transfusion centres:
Medical staff have to notify and counsel donors whose blood is found to be HIV antibody positive.

Specialist AIDS/HIV counsellors have been appointed to deal with the complicated and time-consuming issues in clinical settings.

Who should be Counselled?

Epidemiological studies have identified groups who have been most exposed to HIV infection. When counselling these groups it should be borne in mind that although the incidence of HIV is statistically high, the main risk derives from certain activities and practices. The incidence of AIDS/HIV has spread beyond those groups identified to be at the greatest risk. However, specifically identified 'at risk' groups who might be counselled include:

- Homosexual men
- Bisexual men
- Heterosexual people with several sexual partners
- Intravenous drug users who have shared needles
- Blood and blood product recipients such as haemophiliacs and those who have had blood transfusions before the introduction of routine screening of blood donations
- Those who have had several sexual partners in the last few years, particularly nationals from countries with a high incidence of HIV
- Those who may have been exposed to HIV through certain unhygienic medical and surgical procedures in areas where the seroconversion rate is high
- The sexual partners of all the above groups
- HIV antibody positive mothers
- Health care professionals who have work-related injuries
- All those who perceive themselves to be at risk, for example, people who have been raped, or children who have been sexually abused or assaulted
- People whom the health-care professional perceives to be at risk, such as sexually active teenagers
- Those at all stages of illness related to AIDS/HIV.

Other people who may need counselling

- Those who are apparently well, but who are worried about AIDS/HIV
- The family, the close friends or colleagues of the patient
- Children with HIV and AIDS.

Classification of risk activities in relation to HIV transmission

Considered safe:
Mutual masturbation
Hugging, body rubbing
Massage
Social (dry) kissing
Fantasy
Light sadomasochism (without bleeding or bruising)
Sex toys (when used only on yourself)

Considered possibly safe:
Anal or vaginal intercourse with a condom
French (wet) kissing
Sucking (but stopping before climax)
Urinating on someone
Cunnilingus

Considered unsafe:
Swallowing semen
Anal or vaginal intercourse without a condom
Urinating in the mouth or on skin with sores or cuts
Sharing needles used for intravenous injections
Fisting or rimming
Sharing enema equipment, douching equipment or sex toys

When to Counsel

Counselling begins whenever people express concerns or ask for information. It may also begin when a health care professional perceives a problem. For instance, a doctor may identify the possibility of a risk for HIV when taking the medical history of a woman contemplating pregnancy.

Counselling should be available to patients at different stages of testing, diagnosis and illness. These include:

- Pre- HIV antibody testing
- Post-HIV antibody testing when the result is given and regardless of whether it is negative or positive
- Those who are HIV antibody positive and asymptomatic
- Those who are HIV antibody positive and becoming unwell
- Those with AIDS-related conditions and persistent generalized lymphadenopathy
- Those diagnosed as having AIDS or other major medical conditions which have resulted from HIV infection
- When treatments and investigations are being considered

- When AIDS dementia or neurological impairment is suspected. At such times counselling about how to manage the implications of this condition should be available to the patient, close friends and family
- At times of crisis for the patient or their close contacts
- At the stage of terminal illness when the patient, close contacts and family may have special counselling needs
- After death when relatives, close contacts and others (eg, nurses) may benefit from bereavement counselling
- Those found to be HIV antibody positive in the routine screening of donated blood.

Where to Counsel
The location in which counselling takes place is important because it influences what happens in the session. It is easier to cope with the more frightening aspects of AIDS/HIV in privacy and away from possible interruptions. Counselling may take place at the bedside of an ill patient, in a counselling room, or in the patient's home, and preferably in a pleasant atmosphere. *Conversations in corridors and waiting rooms should be avoided.* Patients may ask critical questions, or raise issues as they are leaving the interview or in unsuitable places because they are either avoiding further discussion or hearing answers to certain questions. This situation can be avoided if the patients' main concerns are addressed early on in the session. The application of this procedure, which includes very close questioning, is described in Chapters 7, 8 and 9.

3
Aims of the counselling session

Most points that are presented in this chapter concern the aims and principles familiar to most professionals already involved in counselling. These are summarized here to refresh the reader's memory.

The Aims of the Session

Each session should provide an opportunity to:

- Talk to the patient
- Listen to what is said and note what is not said
- Identify concerns and help the patient manage them
- Provide information about AIDS/HIV infection
- Assess the psychological and emotional impact of these concerns on the patient
- Assess the behaviour of the patient for possible neurological and psychiatric manifestations of HIV infection
- Consider the relationship difficulties that may emerge between the patient and his contacts and also between the patient and other health care workers
- Assure the patient that his views have been heard
- Help the patient make informed decisions which might influence his behaviour
- Identify the patient's past ways of coping and develop new methods for this if necessary
- Encourage the patient to make decisions and manage his or her life as circumstances permit.

How to Achieve the Aims of Counselling

1. Objectives should be small, limited and attainable
Counsellors can feel overwhelmed by the problems a patient brings to a session. This causes uncertainty and lack of confidence which is easily conveyed to the patient who may then feel even more anxious. To avoid this it is very important to have specific and realizable objectives for each session so that progress can be made and a goal achieved. This might include merely listening to the patient's story or identifying problems where specialized help might be required. If the objectives are clear and attainable the patient may be enabled to manage his difficulties better.

2. The counsellor should lead the session
The counsellor takes the lead in setting up the session, defining its purpose

and guiding the conversation. The content of the interview, that is, what is said, relates to the most pressing concerns of the patient. At the end of the session the patient should feel that he has had an opportunity to talk, explore concerns and have a strategy for dealing with some of them. Listening to the patient is a crucial part of counselling.

3. Assessment

Assessment is continuous and includes the referral material as well as reference to reviews of previous sessions. Since problems and peoples' view of them change over time it is important to identify: (i) a patient's main concern, (ii) his mental state, (iii) what additional resources may be required. In making an assessment the counsellor listens to what is said, how it is said and what might be implied by what is said.

4. Helping the patient to view their problems differently

It is most unlikely that counselling will influence the outcome of a patient's illness, but it can help the patient manage his illness. By challenging existing beliefs counselling can help the patient to view himself and his illness differently. For example, he may realize that his illness has brought him closer to an estranged member of the family. Furthermore a patient who is helped to be more mobile may feel less dependent on others and consequently may then feel less depressed.

5. Reducing anxiety to manageable proportions

Helping the patient manage anxiety can enable him to make decisions and to cope better with his illness. After the counsellor has heard and assessed the patient's problems the first major intervention may be to help him develop a plan for coping with these difficulties. The following is an example of how this might be done:

> **Patient**: I just feel overwhelmed - I don't know what to do next...
> **Counsellor**: What is the most overwhelming aspect for you?
> **Patient**: Everything! Well, maybe how much longer I can get myself to work...
> **Counsellor**: What ideas have you got for when you are unable to manage at work?
> **Patient**: I have a friend who said she'd help me out a bit if I did some work for her at home; but then I get so tired...
> **Counsellor**: If you continue to get so tired and if you were not able to manage anything at all for a while, would you consider sickness benefit?
> **Patient**: I'd be very reluctant to, but then maybe I'd just have to at that point.
> **Counsellor**: Is that something we need to think about now?
> **Patient**: Who would I have to contact?
> (and so on).

As soon as a plan has been developed it is possible to explore the patient's reaction to becoming incapacitated and all the implications of this. Practical management of problems must be dealt with immediately in order to reduce anxiety and also because illness can develop rapidly.

6. Avoiding dependency

Sometimes counsellors are tempted to help by trying to solve the patient's problems. This can lead to the patient becoming overly dependent on the counsellor, which may result in the patient feeling helpless and maybe angry. Many patients have had some form of trauma in their lives, such as the death of someone close, being unemployed or ill, and probably had the capacity to cope without professional help. The counsellor should try to understand how the patient has managed such situations in the past and how these experiences could be used to deal with the present condition. It is important to encourage the patient to realize that he has the capacity to do some things himself as this will help him feel that he has some control over his illness and life.

7. Respecting the patient's own way of coping

Some patients may deny that they are ill or potentially so and the counsellor should respect this as being a way of coping, no matter how irrational it might seem. The counsellor should be guarded against confronting patients who use denial as a coping mechanism as the patient might become very anxious, depressed and possibly suicidal, or totally dependent on the counsellor.

8. Setting boundaries

The counsellor must clearly convey the limits of what can possibly be achieved in the sessions. Confusion over what can and cannot be expected is damaging to the counsellor - patient relationship. If counsellors offer what they cannot in reality provide, they will ultimately let the patient down. For example, the offer of 'you can contact me any time' has to be backed up by a workable plan and the patient must also be told who to contact in case the counsellor is not available. Professional boundaries must be respected otherwise the patient will become too dependent on the counsellor and come to believe that he cannot cope by himself.

9. Assumptions should not be made

It is wise to take nothing for granted and not to make assumptions about the patient's level of knowledge, his concerns, values, and possible reactions, or how he should behave in relationships. Making assumptions inhibits free discussion and exploration of the true nature of the patient's worries. In one case, it was assumed that a university lecturer in psychology understood the meaning of the HIV antibody test result, but it emerged through discussion that he thought his positive HIV antibody result meant that he was protected from AIDS due to the antibodies.

10. Continuity between sessions

It is necessary to regard each session as independent yet connected to the previous meeting so that the patient's major concerns can be continually assessed. For instance, a patient might want to discuss 'safer' sexual activities in one session and how to cope with a disfiguring skin condition in the next.

11. Complete reassurance should not be given

Although research into AIDS/HIV infection has increased our understanding of the nature of the disease, much is still unknown. As a consequence, staff and patients have to find ways of dealing with uncertainty, i.e. information that can be incomplete, conflicting and tentative. The result of this can be that some counsellors may rely on statistics as a way of coping with such uncertainty, but this is of little comfort to patients.

12. Sharing of responsibilities

When necessary, referrals to other specialists should be made as time, resources and expertise are always limited. For example, a patient who is very depressed could be referred to a psychiatrist.

4
The theoretical framework: A lifecycle and developmental approach

AIDS/HIV infection can place considerable stress on family relationships and it is therefore important to take the patient's sexual partners, lovers, and family members into account when trying to find ways of managing the patient's illness, whether they are merely worried about HIV or facing death. Children, siblings, parents and spouses of those who have AIDS/HIV infection should be included, with the patients permission. Our experience of working with AIDS/HIV infected patients has led us to extend the definition of 'family' to include not only those who are related to patients by *birth,* but also those related by *choice.* For example, a homosexual couple may be a family of choice, as may those individuals who provide support and care when the family of origin is unable to do this for one reason or another.

Counselling may focus on the individual patient without ever touching upon the relationship dilemmas that patients with AIDS/HIV infection face. In our experience counsellors can help patients best if they maintain a perspective which takes into account the impact of the patient's illness, behaviour and feelings on those around them. The way in which these people react to the patient at different stages of their illness in turn affects how the patient is able to manage and cope.

A crisis of AIDS is essentially a boundary marker, that is, patients will have to make decisions about who they will continue to have a close relationship with, who they will tell and who they will look to for support. The key dilemma that patients with AIDS/HIV infection face from the counsellor's point of view is the following:

When facing a potentially life-threatening illness most people look to those around them, particularly the family, for support and sustenance. However, some people may always have had a poor relationship with their family or have, through various circumstances, become distant and independent of them. A crisis like AIDS/HIV infection can highlight the patterns of these past relationships with all family members.

Some patients with AIDS/HIV can have unique and specific difficulties when trying to engage the support of their families. This is particularly true if there is anxiety about:

- Becoming stigmatized
- Contaminating others
- Becoming isolated
- Talking about sex and sexuality
- Dying before one's parents

- Parents having to assume a caring role again after children have left home
- Guilt arising from infidelity and promiscuity
- Betrayal
- Secrets between family members
- Secrets between the family and those around them
- Extreme or intense anger between family members
- Issues surrounding death.

There may also be tension if the family is overprotective or, on the other hand, inaccessible and remote. There may be extremes of feelings and reactions between lovers because of the dilemmas they may face. AIDS/HIV infection may incite feelings of intense hatred towards the partner who may have caused a life-threatening infection. It can also strengthen bonds between couples, friends and family members, all of whom may share a similar fate.

Themes that emerge in families where one or more members have a life-threatening illness include:

- Ideas about continuity of the family
- Leaving others behind and being left behind
- How things will be and feel after someone has died.

An important therapeutic task of the counsellor is to help the patient, families and others to get closer (engage) in order to discuss issues which they might find difficult or which might require settlement. In this way they need not part with unfinished business between them.

BACKGROUND TO THE APPROACH

The counselling approach outlined in this book draws on the ideas and techniques of the Milan Associates from the Milan Centre for Family Therapy. The key concepts are:

1. The Systemic View
2. Formulating Hypotheses
3. Using Questions Therapeutically (Circularity)
4. Striving Towards Neutrality

The Systemic View

This view considers the reciprocity of relationships. For instance, if something happens to one member of a family it will affect the rest of the family whose response, in turn, will affect the behaviour of that individual. This means that behaviour cannot be studied in isolation without taking into account the situation in which it occurs. All behaviour is an interactive process whether at home, at work, or in a counselling session. The counsellor may influence the patient whose reactions in turn have an effect on the counsellor. Counselling is not a process of 'doing something to someone'. It is best defined as an interaction between the counsellor and the patient and also includes others such as the patient's family, lovers, friends, and the counsellor's colleagues, as well as members of the health care team.

Counsellors should always take into account the limitations of their particular setting as this determines what it is possible to offer to patients in their day to day care. Broader political and economic issues of the health system will also have to be considered. For example, if a hospital is unable to offer a particular drug that may help AIDS patients, this will determine or at least influence the care of the patients. The counsellor may then have to deal with the frustration and anger of patients who might feel that they are not being offered the full range of possible treatment. This apparent injustice might make people feel bitter and angry.

THE SYSTEMIC VIEW:
INTERACTIONAL COMPLEXITY IN THE COUNSELLING SETTING

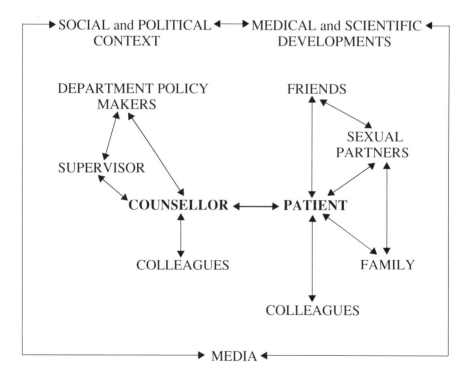

Formulating Hypotheses
An hypothesis, or calculated guess, is made before the session to provide a focus and help the counsellor to begin to address important issues. The following questions are used in formulating a preliminary hypothesis based

on whatever information relating to patients and others (including staff) is available before, during and after the session:

- Why has the patient come to us at this point?
- Who else may be involved, or at least implicated?
- Who else might this session affect?
- What might happen if the counselling session did not take place?
- What is the referrer expecting of the counsellor?
- What stage of life has the patient reached?
- What stage of illness has the patient reached?
- What might the impact be on the referrer if the patient were to improve or deteriorate as a consequence of counselling?
- What are the key issues to be addressed in the session?

Hypotheses may change as they are always conditional and every piece of new information may lead to the revision of ideas.

Using Questions Therapeutically (Circularity)

Questions are used in order to gather information about interactions, patterns of behaviour, relationships and beliefs, and this information is used to link people to each other and to ideas and feelings not often overtly expressed. 'Circularity' is achieved by the use of sequential questions.

A wide range of questions can be asked which have the net effect of helping people to talk about difficult issues and see their situation differently. Ways of coping with and adjusting to circumstances can then be addressed. All questions are potentially therapeutic in so far as hearing the question can challenge a person's ideas and views and each question is designed to gather information about one aspect of a relationship. The use of multiple questions helps to develop a more complete view of relationships, but questions should not lead to a simple 'yes' or 'no' answer because that ends rather than opens up the conversation. Questions are asked that encourage the patient to consider, in the answer, his or her relationship with others.

Questions might address:

- Relationships
- Difficult situations for the management of treatment
- Knowledge about AIDS/HIV infection
- The impact of any of the above on any other person.

There are a number of different questions that can be used. Examples of these are illustrated in the table opposite.

EXAMPLES OF QUESTIONS

Question type	Example
Linear	How do you feel?
Relationship	Who worries more about your becoming ill: your mother or your father? How do they show this? How do you react to them?
Difference	Is it more or less stressful for you to know your T_4-cell test results from month to month?
Circular	How do you imagine it would affect your relationship with her if your wife knew you were coming to this clinic? If I were to ask your boyfriend what his view would be, what do you imagine he would say?
Hypothetical / Future-oriented	If you had to be admitted to hospital as an in-patient, and had not told your boyfriend about your positive antibody test, what might be the effect of this on your relationship? What difficulties might arise for him and for you?

Hypothetical and circular questions are particularly useful when potentially difficult situations need to be addressed. Introducing these questions into counselling interviews has a number of effects:

- Patients and their contacts are helped to view their situation differently which might lead to their finding new ways of coping
- Members of the health care team and related professionals may begin to identify those other people who are likely to support the patient
- 'Dreaded issues' about loss, disfigurement, death and dying can be approached in a way that encourages the patient to talk about them. It is also an indication that the counsellor is not afraid to address these issues with the patient
- Uncertainty can be addressed more easily by asking questions because the counsellor is under less pressure to provide definitive answers
- The counsellor can adopt a more inquisitive style and relax more if a repertoire of questions is developed. This in turn will ease the pressure on the counsellor to find solutions where there may be none. This can help to reduce 'burnout' in staff.

Striving Towards Neutrality

All attempts on the part of the counsellor to preserve a professional relationship, and to resist being distracted and tantalized by any information given by the patient, can help the counsellor to be more neutral and effective.

Neutrality may be achieved if the counsellor respects any view or position that the patient may take. It is probable that the counsellor will have some feeling about what is discussed in the session, but it is another matter as to how the counsellor responds to this. Too many comments designed to comfort and identify with the patient may change the definition from a professional relationship to one of friendship. Statements such as "Oh gosh! How awful for you! I know just what it is to feel like that!" make assumptions about how others feel. Being too friendly defines the relationship in a way that might be difficult to reverse at other times when it might be necessary, such as when having to give bad news.

The counsellor should not have any preconceived ideas about what is best for the patients and what decisions they should make. This does not mean, however, that any behaviour is acceptable even though the counsellor may respect the patient's predicament. For example, a general practitioner who is looking after a family may be concerned about the health of the wife and children of a man who is HIV antibody positive. This man may not want to tell his wife about his condition. The general practitioner may then have to make a decision about whether to inform her of the risk of HIV infection, and how best to do this. Complete neutrality can never be achieved in counselling but the following guidelines may help the counsellor to achieve a balanced stance:

- Being in control of the session without aligning with, or supporting, any particular person or any view presented
- Asking many questions and being interested in the views of patients and their contacts
- Using a neutral tone of voice which does not necessarily convey surprise, astonishment, agreement or anger
- Arranging to ask a colleague to observe the counsellor's interaction with patients. This could mean having a colleague sit in on an interview, or having a discussion with colleagues about the session.

DEVELOPMENTAL FRAMEWORK

No illness occurs in isolation, it affects all those around the patient and this, in turn, depends on the stage of illness the patient has reached. Further, the implications of AIDS/HIV infection in an infant are different from those of an adolescent, a homosexual man, an unmarried 28 years old woman, a blood donor, and so on.

The developmental framework used for counselling patients with AIDS/HIV has three components:

1. The patient's stage of illness in relation to AIDS/HIV infection
2. The patient's stage of development in their own life
3. The stage of development of the individual patient in relation to his own family

The three developmental frameworks are summarized as follows:

Stage of AIDS/HIV	Worried about AIDS
	HIV antibody test
	HIV antibody negative
	HIV antibody positive and asymptomatic
	p24 antigen positive/negative
	HIV antibody positive and symptomatic
	AIDS and AIDS - related illnessess
	Terminal stage of illness
Individual's stage of development	Birth
	Infant
	Child
	Adolescent
	Young adult
	Adult
	Mature adult
	Old age
	Dying
Family's stage of development	Marriage/cohabitation
	Child in family
	Adolescent in family
	Leaving home
	Mid-life
	Divorce/reconstituted family
	Old age
	Death and dying
	Bereavement

This framework helps the counsellor consider:

- What specific issues about HIV infection might be of concern to a patient at a particular age?
- What specific issues about HIV infection might relate currently to this patient in his family?
- What is it about the stage of illness the patient has reached that might help the counsellor address its effect on the patient's family and others? What response in the family can be anticipated if the patient's condition deteriorates?
- What existing problems add to the stress of AIDS/HIV infection?

- Which existing problems are exacerbated by AIDS/HIV infection?
- If the patient did not have AIDS/HIV infection, what other potential problems could arise at this point in their life?

These considerations enable the counsellor to organize information about the similarities and differences between patients. While patients who are diagnosed as having AIDS may have similar concerns, the way they may deal with them, the impact of the diagnosis on them, and even who they choose to tell, will differ from patient to patient.

An application of this frame of reference is outlined in the two examples that follow:

EXAMPLE ONE
Illustrating: (i)   Leaving home problem in the context of a person HIV antibody positive and symptomatic
             (ii)   Young adult
             (iii) Death in the family

A young man of 21 was HIV antibody positive. He had recently left home and come to live in London away from his parents. His relationship with his parents had been tense for the last eighteen months as his parents suspected he was gay, but this had never been openly talked about in the family. His move to London was an attempt to become more independent of his parents and to lead a more 'open' gay life. However, when he first visited the clinic he had been worried about a 'blotch' on his face which the physicians believed to be Kaposi's sarcoma. He was still trying out new relationships, some of which had a sexual component. He felt a marked person, estranged from his family, anxious about how his friends might react and certainly not able to cope with meeting new people.

The approach with this patient was to spend a considerable amount of the counselling time exploring the implications of his homosexuality and illness on the family. He was then helped to find a way of talking to his parents, which was what he most wanted to do. He was anxious that they should not interfere with the way he had chosen to live, or to use his illness as a means to get him to come home and treat him as a child again. The patient took the initiative to telephone his parents to ask them to come to see him in London. He then arranged for his parents to attend a counselling session. The session was used to examine the implications of the illness on each of the parents, and on a younger son, (who had not previously been mentioned by the patient). While there was a great deal of tension in the session, the couple found a way to support their son without having him come home. The relief to everyone was considerable. A further session was planned at their request to help them cope with the social stigma they felt they would have to face as a family. This session also revealed that the patient's younger brother was now doing much better at school. It was hypothesized that the 'secret' in the family and the tension that followed from this had affected his younger brother's progress.

After the patient died, bereavement counselling then helped the parents and their surviving son cope with and adjust to their loss.

EXAMPLE TWO
Illustrating: (i) Mature adult worried about AIDS
   (ii) Children leaving home
   (iii) Marriage difficulties and divorce

A man of 54 made an appointment to see a counsellor as he was worried he might have contracted AIDS. Through the pre-test counselling session it emerged that he was married with two children, aged 24 and 21. He had had several sexual encounters with other men over the last two years. No one in the family was aware of his bisexuality. In the session it was discussed what it would mean for him if he were HIV antibody positive, if his wife and children were to find out about his bisexuality, and the implications for all of them if he were to become unwell. He then stated that his marriage had not been good for at least five years, and now that both his children had moved away from home he had to spend more time with his wife. He had started to use work as an excuse for coming home late.

It was hypothesized that the children's leaving home had aggravated his mid-life crisis and an unsettled marriage. He had found his sexual enjoyment outside the marriage as a means of revitalizing himself and avoiding his wife. A recent media campaign, coupled with his own guilt, had forced him to make a decision about his marriage. The threat of HIV infection and coming for the test was a point of crisis. The counsellor was able to explore how the result might influence his decision about the marriage. He was later referred for the test. He had been protecting his wife from possible infection by not sleeping with her for the last two years and he agreed not to change this until there could be some confirmation of his HIV antibody status. He was found to be HIV antibody negative and arrangements were made for him to have another test in three months time. What followed from this was that he told his wife that he wanted to leave her. He had discussed with the counsellor how he might do this. His greatest fear was how she might react, and that she might not agree to a separation as he no longer wanted to keep his bisexuality a secret. During the counselling session he discussed various ways of approaching his wife, and how he might deal with her reactions. He managed to tell his wife, and she wanted to have the HIV antibody test herself. They continued to see the counsellor together to renegotiate how to continue their relationship in the future as his wife did not want a divorce.

THE HEALTH CARE TEAM: A DEVELOPMENTAL APPROACH
A final aspect of the developmental approach is the development of the services for patients with AIDS/HIV infection. To illustrate this, the hospital-based health care team will be referred to (see Chapter 10).

Each team has a different history and unique management considerations.

Approaches to the care of patients with AIDS/HIV infection are not uniform. This is not to suggest that there are different standards of care but, rather, different approaches to care. These are influenced by unit, local district and national forces, some of which may be at variance with one another. Another source of influence is the cumulative knowledge about the history and epidemiology of HIV infection. Before 1988, there might have been less reason to test for antibodies to HIV because there was little that could be done for patients. From a medical point of view, there are increased advantages of knowing the HIV antibody status of patients: there is more widespread use of antiviral drugs since 1987 and medical surveillance makes it possible to diagnose and treat symptoms early.

Developments in medical and allied fields have had an important impact on the content and process of what happens in the counselling situation. How each unit assimilates and uses these developments may differ.

For this reason, the counsellor has to respond to the patient's difficulties in an ever-evolving treatment environment, extending from the particular hospital, unit or surgery to the rapid advances in medical therapeutics and prevention.

5
Guidelines for the counselling session

The counsellor should be guided by a structure and purpose for each session. The structure gives some form to the session. Decisions have to be made about:

- Who should come to the session
- How much time is available for the session
- How the time will be used (see the guidelines below and Chapter 3)

If care is taken, at the start, to describe, briefly, the purpose and structure of the session, this communicates several points to the patient:

- The counsellor will lead the session
- The counsellor will take an interest in the patient's problems and will help to develop ideas on how to deal with them
- It is a planned session focussing on certain identified problems

This is important given the multitude of problems and the intense and emotional response of many patients. In addition, a structure helps the counsellor use the time efficiently and not be overwhelmed by the patient's problems. If there is no structure the net result may be that the most severe problems are not dealt with during the session and the patient may complain of feeling depressed and make statements such as: "My brain is in such a muddle".

Counselling sessions may be with:

Individuals
Couples
Families
Groups

Guidelines for the Session:

- The patient should be encouraged to bring close contacts or family members to sessions whenever appropriate as this helps in addressing the impact of the patient's illness on others. It also helps to give the counsellor a fuller picture of the patient's circumstances

- The counsellor should develop a hypothesis regarding what the concerns and relationship problems might be just before the session starts.

This helps to guide the interview in order to address the main concerns, and develop ideas on how to cope with them. When developing an initial hypothesis it is useful to consider the following:

(a) **The context** It makes a difference if patients are seen in a general practitioner's surgery, a genitourinary medicine clinic, or at the bedside. If patients come to an genitourinary medicine clinic they may already acknowledge some sexual risk. If a general practitioner detects enlarged lymph glands and oral candidiasis in the course of a routine examination, the subject of AIDS/HIV may have to be broached.

(b) **The referral** It is important to know who made the referral and why the referral was made now; also, what the main concern of the referrer was and what did he hope to achieve by referring the patient? A hidden concern of some referrers may be, for example, their own reluctance to discuss a diagnosis of AIDS with the patient. The referral at this point reflects more the anxiety of the referrer than the patient's problem. An example of a discussion with a referrer follows:

Counsellor: Dr James, what is it you would most want me to discuss with your patient?
Dr James: Well, I haven't yet told him he has AIDS, but I think you could give him some support.
Counsellor: What kind of support would you see me giving that would help you to tell him he has AIDS?

(c) **The patient.** Information about the patient's age, life stage, sex and diagnosis is important. The counsellor should try to answer the question: "What is happening to the patient right now in relation to his or her illness and how might it affect others around them?"

At the beginning of the first session counsellors should:
• Introduce themselves, state their professional background, if appropriate, and mention how they relate to the referrer
• Clarify with the patient how much time is available for the session and indicate what follow-up there might be to the session
• Stress the confidential nature of the interview
• Use questions to help to bring into focus patients' major concerns and their expectations of each session.

Questions help to keep a focus. For example:

Counsellor: If I was to ask you what your main concern is today, what might it be?
Patient: AIDS!

Counsellor: Where does AIDS rank with your other concerns?
Patient: It's the main one.
Counsellor: What is your main concern about AIDS now? (and so on).

- It is important to check in stages what people know about AIDS/HIV before correcting misinformation, and giving new information. This helps to move at the patient's pace and to assess and adapt to his level of understanding. This approach is helpful in addressing both information, relationship and behaviour issues.
  The following sequence can guide the questioning:

Questions about knowledge:
Counsellor: What do you know about the HIV antibody test?

Assessing the source of knowledge:
Counsellor: Where do you get your information from about the
                meaning of the HIV antibody test result?

Correcting misinformation:
Counsellor: No, it is not a test for AIDS.

Addressing the implications of knowledge:
Counsellor: Knowing that you are HIV antibody positive, how does
                this effect your relationship with your lover?

- The counsellor reflects on the patient's last sentence and uses the patient's own words to form the next question. The advantages of this for the counsellor are:

(a) The session moves at the patient's own pace.
(b) A bond between the counsellor and the patient is encouraged.
    For example,when talking to a teenager about condoms, use the slang of 'jonny' or 'rubber'.
(c) A focus is maintained and themes and topics are developed as they emerge.
(d) Patients realize that they have been heard.
(e) The counsellor is able to take time to think about what to say next.
    The use of the patient's own work helps to form a connection between ideas and different people. For example:

Patient: I feel so worried.....
Counsellor: What is it that worries you the most?
Patient: That my parents will be upset when they hear the news.
Counsellor: What news is it that you think will upset them?
Patient: That our general practitioner knows I am gay and he is a family friend.

Counsellor: Knowing this, how might it affect your general
practitioner's relationship with your parents? (and so on).

Throughout the interview the counsellor should endeavour to make a
link with the patient between **information, behaviour, relationships**
and **beliefs.**

The following diagram illustrates how this can be done:

A. INFORMATION/STATEMENTS

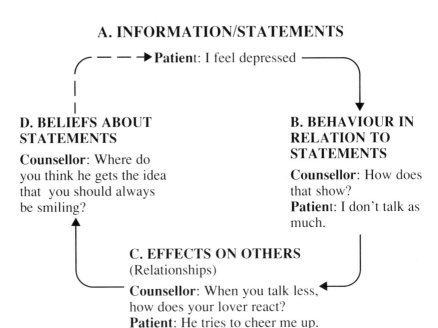

Patient: I feel depressed

**D. BELIEFS ABOUT
STATEMENTS**

Counsellor: Where do
you think he gets the idea
that you should always
be smiling?

**B. BEHAVIOUR IN
RELATION TO
STATEMENTS**

Counsellor: How does
that show?
Patient: I don't talk as
much.

C. EFFECTS ON OTHERS
(Relationships)

Counsellor: When you talk less,
how does your lover react?
Patient: He tries to cheer me up.

- Using a neutral, enquiring tone of voice conveys respect for whatever is said. The counsellor is then less likely to influence what the
  patient talks about. The advantages of this have been discussed in
  Chapter 4.
  In order to help keep the interview focused and to be as neutral and
  objective as possible the counsellor might include a colleague, such
  as a nurse or a doctor, in the session. The person who is not actively
  interviewing can help the counsellor to be more objective and
  creative. In addition, they may also challenge the views of the
  counsellor, which, in turn, may increase the number of ideas and
  possibilities that can emerge from the session.

- The counsellor should always pay attention to both the content and
  the process: that is, what is said (or not said), and how it is said or
  conveyed. If a patient keeps telephoning the counsellor in order to

talk, but resists taking up the invitation to meet personally for a session, the counsellor might make the hypothesis that the patient prefers to keep a distance and might have difficulty facing up to some issue. Observation and assessment of behaviour is a central component of counselling. It is of particular importance in AIDS counselling where patients may be developing neurological impairment or may show evidence of psychiatric symptoms.

- It is useful for the counsellor to take a break just before the end of the session. This can be done in various ways:
  – By leaving the room and returning after a brief interval. The counsellor might reflect alone, or discuss some of the ideas with a colleague.
  – By staying in the room, or at the bedside, and recapitulating what has been said, without discussion, until the summary of thoughts and ideas is complete.

This break can help the counsellor to reflect on what has happened in the session, and to gain some emotional distance. Furthermore, it provides an opportunity for the counsellor to revise his views of the patient. In this way, patients are given a more considered opinion about how the counsellor sees they are managing with AIDS/HIV. This break also helps the patient to collect their own ideas and thoughts and to have some distance from some of the issues being talked about.

Here is a list of some questions that counsellors might ask of themselves or a colleague when reviewing a session. The answers may guide the counsellor's thoughts about how to handle the case:

QUESTIONS IN REVIEWING A CASE

What is the problem?
How is it defined? By whom?
What does the patient expect of me in relation to the problem?
Why does this problem appear at this point in time?
Who else is implicated?
What stage of life has the patient reached?
What would happen if the situation deteriorated?
- to the patient?
- to the referrer?
- to the friends and family of the patient?
- to the counsellor?
Why is the patient telling me this?
How is the patient telling me this?
Who else is the patient telling?
Who else should the patient be telling?

> How can I best deal with the problem?
> What is the worst possible consequence of what the patient is
>   telling me?
> How do I feel about it?
> What is the explicit message? Implicit message?
> What are the settings in which all this takes place?
> What is the least that needs to be done in order to bring
>   about a change?
> How does the patient (partner) view me at present?
> What behaviour tells me that this is how the patient feels?
> If my colleagues were in here now, what might they advise
>   me to do?

- A future follow-up appointment should be given at the end of most sessions. If this is not arranged, there should be a clear statement about the end of the counselling contact. Knowing that they have another appointment can help a patient feel supported and more secure as further issues will be discussed. Often, there is insufficient time to adequately explore or develop all the major concerns that arise in any one session. As the illness progresses, so patients will have new concerns that will need to be discussed. If patients leave with the knowledge that there is a future opportunity they may not feel the necessity to telephone or come unexpectedly for appointments. This in turn helps to reduce pressure on staff.

- The time between and the frequency of follow-up appointments is also important. The frequency of sessions depends on each individual situation. Someone awaiting an HIV antibody test result, or an individual who is extremely anxious, may have to be seen more frequently, but for shorter sessions. It is important therapeutically for the impact of a counselling session to have time to take effect. Meetings which are too frequent are a communication to patients that they cannot cope alone. A month is a reasonable span of time while people are well. Once they become ill the length of time between sessions may be reduced, as necessary.

6
The clinical aspects of AIDS/HIV

by
Dr Christine Lee
Consultant Haematologist
Haemophilia Centre,
Royal Free Hospital,
London

In 1981 cases of *Pneumocystis carinii* pneumonia occurring together with Kaposi's sarcoma were reported in young men in America. These were the first recognized cases of the acquired immune deficiency syndrome or AIDS. It was soon realized that these patients were immunocompromised and, co-incidentally, predominantly homosexual. However, it was not until 1983 that the virus known to cause AIDS was discovered. The virus is now called the human immunodeficiency virus or HIV.

Immunological aspects
The human immunodeficiency virus is a retrovirus. It is an RNA virus with a viral enzyme, reverse transcriptase, which allows it to make a DNA copy of its own RNA genetic material. This means that once the RNA viral genome (genetic core) becomes DNA, it can be incorporated into the host cell. The protein of the genetic core is p24 and the main enveloping glyco-proteins are gp 41 and gp120.

The clinical features of HIV infection are a consequence of the immune deficit which occurs with the 'take over' of mainly helper T (thymus derived) lymphocytes. These are a subset of T lymphocytes which have a receptor called CD 4 to which the envelope glycoprotein of HIV will bind. This results in the destruction of T_4 (or helper/inducer lymphocytes) which have a large number of CD4 receptors on the surface. The virus can also enter the genome of the lymphocyte and self-replicate. The T_4 lymphocytes play an important role in the immune response and it is their destruction which accounts for the immunodeficiency effect of the virus. The T_4 lymphocytes divide on antigen-tic stimulation and produce lymphokines or growth factors, one of which is called interleukin 2. The growth factors promote B lymphocyte growth and antibody production. Growth factors also control the growth of T_8 or cytotoxic/suppressor T lymphocytes and tissue macrophages (the macroph-ages are antigen-presenting cells). The changes in the immune system produced by the virus can be demonstrated in man and in the laboratory. Soon after infection, in common with other virus infections, there is an increase in the T_8 or suppressor lymphocytes. There is a reduction in cell-mediated immune responses as shown by an anergy in skin tests to common recall antigens, for example, diphtheria, tuberculin or candida. Antibody to HIV appears three weeks to three months after exposure, but the titre of neutralizing antibody is low. There is a non-specific stimulation of B cells which results in an increase in serum immunoglobulins. The marker of disease progression is a fall in the number of the helper/inducer T_4 lymphocytes. The neutropenia, anaemia, thrombocytopenia and lymphopenia which occurs in infected individuals may have an autoimmune aetiology.

At the time of acute infection and the stimulation of antibodies with HIV, there may be acute seroconversion illness. This can be similar to glandular fever with fever, malaise, muscle aches, joint pains, swollen lymph glands (lymphadenopathy) and sore throat. However, the acute infection can be asymptomatic.

Lymphadenopathy and AIDS-related complex

After a patient has 'seroconverted' he may progress to chronic infection. During this period minor opportunistic infections may occur, for example, herpes zoster. There may be skin conditions such as seborrhoeic dermatitis and hairy leukoplakia. Lymphadenopathy is often seen during chronic infection and this is known as persistent generalized lymphadenopathy (PGL). It has been defined as enlarged lymph nodes greater than one cm in diameter which occur in two or more sites outside the inguinal areas and this lymphadenopathy should persist for at least three months. The lymph nodes show benign follicular hyperplasia and, on special staining, have been shown to be infiltrated with T_8 lymphocytes and to be depleted of T_4 lymphocytes.

Before the development of end-stage disease, patients may have constitutional symptoms. The AIDS-related complex or ARC has been diagnosed in a patient where two or more signs/symptoms have been present for three months or longer with any two or more abnormal laboratory values. The signs and symptoms include: fever, weight loss, persistent generalized lymphadenopathy, diarrhoea, fatigue and night sweats. The laboratory values include: lymphopenia, leucopenia, thrombocytopenia, anaemia, reduced T_4 : T_8 ratio, reduced T_4 helper cells, raised gammaglobulins, reduced lymphocyte transformation and cutaneous allergy. The usefulness of identifying patients with constitutional disease is that these patients may become particularly ill and progress to fullblown AIDS.

Clinical manifestations of AIDS

The clinical manifestations of fullblown AIDS are a series of opportunistic infections and tumours. The commonest opportunistic infection is *Pneumocystis carinii* pneumonia and pneumonia can also be caused by unusual bacteria, for example, mycobacteria or TB, viruses such as *Cytomegalovirus* (CMV) and fungi such as *Cryptococcus*. These organisms can also affect the central nervous system. In the gut the infecting organisms may be those which primarily infect animals and include the protozoa *Cryptosporidium,* the viruses CMV and herpes, fungi (predominantly *Candida)* and unusual bacteria, for example atypical mycobacteria. The commonest tumour which has been described in AIDS is Kaposi's sarcoma, but non-Hodgkin's lymphoma and squamous carcinomas of the mouth and anorectum also occur.

Pneumonia

The lungs are commonly affected in AIDS and 85 per cent of pulmonary infections are due to *Pneumocystis carinii* pneumonia.Patients present with a dry cough and breathlessness often of some weeks duration. There is invariably fever. The chest X-ray shows diffuse bilateral shadowing. The diagnosis can be confirmed by bronchoalveolar lavage when the cysts of *Pneumocystis carinii* can be demonstrated in the washings. The treatment is high dose Septrin (co-trimoxazole) and, because this may cause severe bone-marrow depression, folinic acid is also given. Many patients progress to respiratory failure and thus mechanical ventilation may be considered. However, the results of mechanical ventilation in this situation are very poor, few patients who survive are alive at one year. Ideally, a discussion about ventilation should be held with the patient before he becomes seriously ill. About 7 per cent of patients survive are first episode of *Pneumocystis carinii*, and in the UK their subsequent life expectancy is 12.5 months.

Kaposi's sarcoma

A diagnosis of AIDS is also made if a patient who is HIV antibody seropositive develops Kaposi's sarcoma or a high grade lymphoma. Kaposi's sarcoma is a malignant tumour which arises from vascular endothelium. It is multifocal and occurs predominantly in the skin or gastrointestinal tract. Before the advent of AIDS, Kaposi's sarcoma was seen on the legs of elderly patients, particularly males of Jewish or East European extraction. Its occurrence in association with AIDS suggests a possible viral aetiology, perhaps a further opportunistic infection. It is of interest that Kaposi's sarcoma is seen much less commonly in association with AIDS secondary to blood or blood product transfusion or intravenous drug abuse. Treatment is difficult. Irradiation has been used especially to prevent the infective hazard of bleeding lesions on the hands and feet. High-dose interferon has also been used, but this has very severe side-effects of shivering, fevers and general malaise. Often local cosmetic application is helpful where there are facial lesions.

Lymphoma

Malignant lymphoma is the second most common malignant tumour which affects patients who have AIDS. The lymphoma often presents at an advanced stage with symptoms of fever and weight loss. The lymphoma is present in extranodal areas: the central nervous system, the bone marrow, the gastrointestinal tract including the mouth, and the skin. The lymphomas are commonly high-grade B cell tumours. Cytotoxic therapy is probably only advisable if the symptoms of lymphoma occur before opportunistic infections. Median survival of patients who have been treated with cytotoxic therapy is usually less than a year.

Candidiasis

Although biopsy - or culture - proven oesophageal candidiasis is required for the diagnosis of AIDS, oral candidiasis alone also indicates a poor prognosis and there is a high risk of the later development of fullblown AIDS. Oral candidiasis is often asymptomatic, but there may be a sore mouth and sore throat. Retrosternal chest pain occurs when there is oesophageal candidiasis and there is often difficulty with swallowing.

Neurological manifestations
The neurological manifestations of AIDS may be due to opportunistic infections, tumours or the direct effect of HIV. The fungus *Cryptococcus neoformans* is the most common cause of meningitis in patients with AIDS. Patients present with headache and the diagnosis is made by India ink staining of the cerebrospinal fluid (CSF) or by detecting the cryptococcal antigen in the serum or CSF. Headache is also a major presenting complaint of patients with cerebral toxoplasmosis. There is usually a focal neurological lesion and the CT scan will show mass lesions. Similar CT scan appearances are shown where there are abscesses caused by infection with *Candida albicans* or *Mycobacterium tuberculosis*. Cytomegalovirus causes a retinitis and this is the most common cause of impaired visual acuity in patients with AIDS. On ophthalamic examination, the retinal vessels are narrowed and there are exudates and haemorrhages around vessels. Ultimately, areas of the retina are infarcted and this leads to blindness. Space-occupying lesions can be caused by opportunistic infections, for example, the protozoon *Toxoplasma gondii,* or tumours. Such lesions present with focal neurological lesions or fits.

The human immunodeficiency virus can produce primary neurological defects and these can occur in immunocompetent people who are HIV antibody positive. The receptor for HIV, the CD4 molecule, occurs predominantly on T_4 lymphocytes. However, its distribution is much wider and it occurs on CNS microglial cells. In this situation the virus may be directly cytopathic. Clinically, the AIDS dementia complex may start with cognitive changes of memory loss, impaired concentration, mental slowing and confusion. There may be behavioural changes of apathy, 'depression' or withdrawal. Sometimes behaviour is hyperactive with agitation, confusion or even hallucinations. Motor changes include unsteadiness of gait, leg weakness, loss of co-ordination manifested by impaired handwriting and tremor. The illness can progress rapidly to dementia within weeks or months. Terminally, the neurological disease can result in the patient being bedridden and incontinent. The CT scan shows cerebral atrophy which is particularly obvious in a young person. The neuropathological change occurs in the central white matter with sparing of the cortex.

Testing for HIV
The most widely used test for HIV is a test for antibody. Anti-HIV appears three weeks to three months after exposure to HIV. However, some individuals have extremely low concentrations of anti-HIV, particularly early in infection, and such low levels may not be detected. HIV can be produced in cell lines in order to provide antigen for serological tests. Most tests use as an end-point the colour reaction of an enzyme and substrate. The antibody

to HIV present in a test serum binds to HIV antigen fixed to the base of a well in a test plate. Immunoglobulin linked to the enzyme will then bind to the HIV antigen-antibody complex. This type of test is referred to as an ELISA, enzyme linked immunoabsorbent assay.

Western blot method

A different type of test, but one which also measures HIV antibody, is the Western blot method. Disrupted HIV virus (which has been produced in cell lines) is separated into different antigenic components by electrophoresis on a polyacrylamide gel. HIV antibody which may be present in the test serum can be blotted onto the viral antigens. An antigen-antibody complex of HIV can then be demonstrated using a radiolabelled antihuman immunoglobulin. Using such a technique it is possible to recognize different components of the antibody response. It may also be possible to differentiate the earlier IgM anti-HIV response which precedes the IgG response. Since the finding of antibody to HIV has such profound consequences, it is vital to ensure accurate testing. Repeat testing by an anti-HIV test which uses different methodology is advised in the UK when there is a positive anti-HIV result. Although this has a problem of delay it does give precision.

Testing for p24

More recently, testing for the main HIV core antigen (p24) has become available. This is detectable where there is an excess of antigen over antibody to p24.

This occurs at the time of infection and also in advanced infection. Thus, 70 per cent of patients with AIDS have detectable p24. It is possible that the p24 antigen may be helpful as a predictor of the increased risk of subsequent AIDS in anti-HIV seropositive patients. It was also hoped that measurement of the p24 antigen would be helpful in providing an indication for, and assessing the subsequent effectiveness of antiviral therapy. However, since the p24 antigen is not detected in 30 per cent of patients with AIDS its use is clearly limited.

Treatment

The treatment of AIDS has mostly involved the treatment of opportunistic infections and tumours. Specific antiviral agents have been and are being developed for use in man. The targets for antiviral therapy are at the point of entry to the cell: the binding to the CD4 receptor, the translation of viral RNA to DNA: the enzyme reverse transcriptase, and the sites of viral replication and viral budding. An ideal drug should provide a number of features. It should protect uninfected cells, reduce viral production, be orally absorbed, penetrate the CSF and have low toxicity. AZT, 3' azido 3' deoxythymidine, is the first drug which has been shown to be beneficial for patients with AIDS and is the drug which is currently undergoing much study in patients. AZT is a dideoxynucleoside analogue, acting as a chain terminator of DNA during reverse transcription. As soon as the enzyme reverse transcriptase has been fooled into adding the nucleoside to the growing chain of DNA, no subsequent nucleosides can be added and the DNA chain is terminated. It is of interest that AZT was first synthesized 20 years ago and was shown over 12 years ago to inhibit replication of C-type murine retrovirus. The drug has been shown to improve immunological function and HIV- related neurological abnormality. Overall, patients receiving AZT have lived longer than controls. The main problem is the drug's depression of bone marrow requiring frequent blood tranfusions to maintain haemoglobin levels. A number of other antiviral agents have been produced: phosphonoformate inhibits reverse transcriptase and although it has reduced viral replication in small controlled trials, it has the disadvantage of requiring intravanous administration; ribavirin is a guanine analogue which prevents RNA assembly and has had limited success in clinical trials; interferon has been used in the treatment of Kaposi's sarcoma and HIV-related thrombocytopenia. It is probable that in the future there will be combinations of antiviral therapy which will be used in a similar way to anticancer chemotherapy.

The most tantalizing possibility is that of vaccine development. Unfortunatly it is still not clear which of the immune responses to HIV are important for protection. The approach towards the development of a vaccine can either involve immunization using virus antigens or the development of antibodies to the CD4 receptor molecule. Testing of vaccines is difficult because HIV only causes AIDS in man.

The importance of HIV infection and AIDS is not only its high mortality and thus the urgent clinical problem, but also there has never been a disease process which has produced so many complex social issues. Counselling is a most valuable therapeutic tool - certainly until safe, effective drug therapy and vaccination become practicable.

7
The counselling interview: Information and questions

This chapter describes what might be discussed in a clinical counselling session. It is not, however an example of a complete session. Examples of questions are provided for the counsellor in order to begin the conversation. What is included, and how this is done, depends on several factors (see also Chapters 3, 4 and 5):

- The stage of the patient's illness
- His current concerns
- The patient's age, physical and mental state
- What is happening in the patient's relationships
- The setting in which counselling takes place
- New knowledge or treatments relating to AIDS/HIV infection
- Issues currently topical in the media in relation to AIDS/HIV infection
- Techniques and experience of the counsellor.

The following is a list of the essential points that are covered in the chapter:

The issues raised in this left hand column may be discussed during clinical counselling sessions.

The questions raised in this right hand column are designed to help the counsellor to address the issues in the left hand column. This includes questions that can be used for:
  • *Checking knowledge*
  • *Challenging views*

I. MEDICAL ISSUES

Questions to patients

The essential knowledge about Human Immunodeficiency Virus and Acquired Immuno-deficiency Syndrome

"What do you understand about AIDS and HIV?"
"What is your source of information?"

Transmission
This is mainly through sexual activities; exposure to blood and blood products; needle sharing among drugs users; also, mother to unborn child perinatally

"How might the virus be passed on to others?"
"Which sexual activities are considered risky?"

Incubation
There is a long period from infection to developing AIDS
It is unknown whether all those infected will develop AIDS
The percentage of people developing AIDS could increase over time
It is uncertain how long it may take to develop AIDS

"What do you think your chances are of developing AIDS?"
"What do you know about the length of time it might take to develop AIDS?"

"How might you handle the different views and statistics about this?"

It is a retrovirus
Which means it can insert itself into the host cell nucleus
It is sensitive to heat and is easily killed by common sterilizing agents such as bleach

"What do you understand by a 'retrovirus'?"
"Do you have any idea how this virus reproduces itself?"
"Do you know how the virus might be destroyed?"

HIV is infectious:
Once a person is infected it is thought the virus will remain in the body for life.
It is now thought likely that people are more infectious as they become ill

"What is your understanding of how long the virus remains in the body?"
"What do you know about your capacity to infect others over time?"

The 'window period'
Following infection there is a period ranging from about 6 weeks to 3 months, or even longer, before antibodies to HIV can be detected. During the 'window period' the person can be infectious and pass on HIV to others

"When, in your view, was your most recent exposure to HIV?"
"What do you know about the period of being infected and showing a positive antibody to HIV?"
"Does this mean that if we tested you now and you were negative that you could not pass on the virus?"

The process of developing antibodies is called seroconversion. It can be accompanied by a glandular fever-like illness lasting 3-14 days or, rarely, a neurological illness like meningitis
If people are considered to be 'at risk', tests should be repeated after 6, 12 and 18 months

"Is there anyone at risk at the moment?"

"How might you deal with this as there is still uncertainty?"

"Would you be prepared to be tested again?"
"How will you protect yourself and others during this period of uncertainty?"

The HIV antibody test
The test is specific to HIV.
It is an antibody detection test.
The results are checked by a confirmatory test and a second sample
It is not a test for AIDS or the virus.
It is not a diagnosis
It cannot specifically indicate when, or for how long, there has been infection with HIV
The antibodies to HIV are not necessarily protection from developing AIDS

"What do you understand by the HIV antibody test?"
"How reliable do you understand the test to be?"

"Do you think it is a test for AIDS?"
"What information does the result of this test give us?"

"Do you think having the antibodies to HIV protects you from developing AIDS?"

A positive HIV antibody test:
Confirms past infection with HIV
The person is presumed to be infectious and infected for life.
It does not predict with any certainty that the person will develop AIDS

"What do you understand by being HIV antibody positive?"
"Do you think anyone is at risk of being infected by you?"
"What do you know about how long you will remain HIV seropositive?"

A negative HIV antibody test:
Antibodies to the virus have not been detected

"The result is negative. Do you think you should be retested in 3 months time in order to confirm this?"
"As your HIV antibody is negative and you considered there was a risk of infection, when was your last identified risk?"

This may be because seroconversion has not yet taken place - ie, antibodies have not yet been developed. Some people who are infected fail to produce antibodies to HIV

"With this result how will you protect yourself and others in the future?"

The HIV antigen test

This test can identify p24 core antigen of the virus.
The test detects the virus.
In some people with acute infections at the time of seroconversion, p24 can be detected before the development of antibodies. Therefore, a person can be infected with HIV without HIV antibodies being detected. This is referred to as the 'window period'
Positive HIV antigen suggests replication of the virus and the possible depletion of T_4 cells
Antigen tests may have prognostic value and thus be of use to clinicians prescribing antiviral therapy

"Do you know what p24 antigen is?"
"What do you know about the antigen test, and the meaning of a positive result?"
"Knowing that you are antigen positive, what does this mean to you?"

"Is there anything that might have started the virus reproducing itself like an infection?"
"If you were told your antigen results were positive, and the clinicians were considering antiviral therapy, what would be your views?"

Predictive values

Predictive values such as the HIV antibody, p24 antigen and T_4 tests can help clinicians:
  • Make a diagnosis
  • Define the stage and possible out-come of HIV illness
  • Decide when to broach difficult issues with patients
If the meaning of these predictive values is discussed at an appropriate, early stage the patient may be better prepared to make decisions about his life

"What do you understand about these routine tests?"
"Do you want to be informed about the results of tests?"
"In what way would knowing these results help you?"
"Are there any ways that knowing the results might make it more difficult for you?"

The immune system

HIV targets itself at the immune system.

HIV can result in a person becoming susceptible to a group of opportunistic infections and virus-associated tumours. This clinical condition is called acquired immunodeficiency syndrome, AIDS

HIV destroys the immune cells in blood and tissues - the T_4 lymphocytes

HIV virus replication can be stimulated by intercurrent infections

Some co-factors that might stimulate virus replication are:

(i) Other sexually transmitted diseases

(ii) Pregnancy in an HIV seropostive woman

(iii) Poor health: a poor diet, unremitting stress and insufficient sleep and exercise do not enhance the functioning of the immune system.

"What does AIDS stand for?"

"Do you know what the function of the immune system is?"
"Do you know how HIV interferes with the immune system?"

"Do you know what might increase your chance of developing infections?"
"What steps can you take to avoid getting other sexually transmitted diseases?"

"What do you know about the effect of pregnancy on your own health if you are antibody positive?"
"What do you think you might do to keep well?"

Symptoms of AIDS

Some of the most common are:

- Palpable and enlarged lymph glands
- Fatigue
- Dyspnoea/breathlessness
- Dry cough
- Fever
- Loss of weight
- Diarrhoea
- Some skin conditions
- Night sweats

"What is it that made you decide to come here today?"
"What symptoms do you think are important for the doctor to check?"
"How long has this been troubling you?"
"Have you had an HIV test?"
"Have you had any treatment and what effect did it have?"
"Are you asking me whether you have moved on from being asymptomatic and whether these might be symptoms of AIDS?"

Many symptoms are similar to those of acute anxiety and depression
Patients need to be aware of some of the symptoms which might respond to prompt treatment.

"Why do you think it is important to have regular check-ups by your doctor?"
"What do you know about the treatment of this infection?"
"If you developed any symptoms or thought you were becoming unwell what would you do and who might you tell?"
"How long would you wait before consulting a doctor?"
"Would you contact your general practitioner or the clinic?"

Antiviral and other treatments
Known side-effects of treatment should be discussed whenever possible
If the patient is part of a clinical trial, or if treatment involves frequent surveillance it is essential to ascertain the patient's willingness and ability to co-operate. This might mean frequent attendance at the hospital or general practitioners' surgeries

"What do you know about the possibility of treatment?"
"What do you know about the side-effects?"
"What do you know about the outcome of such treatment?"
"If you were to be offered treatment or to be part of a clinical trial would you be able to attend frequently?"
"If you were in my position as a doctor and you needed to take blood monthly from a patient as part of giving treatment but he was unwilling to come back, how would you handle this?"

Vaccines
Vaccines for HIV are being developed but are not yet available
People ask about them and who will or should be given such a vaccine
Vaccines against other illnesses: Polio, chicken pox etc.
Live vaccines are not recommended for those with HIV

"What do you know about the availability of a vaccine?"

"Who do you think should be given vaccines if they were available?"
"What do you know about the use of vaccines, live or dead, if you have HIV?"
"What might be the risks or the benefits?"
"Are you likely to move into a job or travel where you might be required to have a vaccination?"

Clinical care of patients

Issues that may need clarification include:

- How to get medical care
- Who has principal responsibility for looking after the patient

- Where should care be offered

"What are your views about how you would like to get medical care?"

"If you feel unwell, or you have some questions to ask, will you come here to the hospital or go to your general practitioner first?"

"It is not clear whether you want your general practitioner or the hospital to organize your care."

"What would your views be about being admitted to an AIDS ward if hospitalization became necessary?"

"If you were very ill and there was an option of being cared for at home or in hospital which would you prefer?"

Confidentiality

Who to tell.

Who *should* be told, such as:

- General practitioner
- Community nurse
- Dentist

How information is passed on

- Verbally
- In a letter

"Who would you like to tell about your HIV status?"

"Who do you think ought to know?"

"If on telling your dentist he refuses to treat you, what might you do?"

"Have you thought about telling your general practitioner but asking him not to write it in your notes?"

"What is it in your relationship with your general practitioner that makes you decide not to tell her?"

Encourage patients to share information with other health care professionals

"We understand that confidentiality is very important. Sometimes, for your benefit, other professionals need to be included in your care. Do you have any objection to them being told when necessary?"

"If your general practitioner was not told you had HIV how might this affect your care?"

Some patients give double messages about whether they want to be informed about bad news or not. It can be difficult for health care professionals to know what to say and when it should be said.

Discuss life-support measures such as resuscitation and ventilation at appropriate times when the patient is still well. Discuss possible neurological manifestations of HIV infection.

"How will we know what information you want? Will this change over time?"
"You complain that staff are not telling you everything. How can you get them to be more open with you?"
"If you were so ill that you needed to be resuscitated or ventilated, what would your views be about this?"
"If you were unable to make decisions for yourself who would you want to make them for you?"

Transmission and prevention of HIV
Discuss how the virus is transmitted and clarify 'true risk'

a) Sexual transmission:
  • Man to man
  • Man to woman
  • Woman to man

b) The risk activities :
See Chapter 2

"What is your understanding of how the HIV is transmitted, or passed on?"
"What do you mean by 'sex'? Is it kissing, hugging etc...?"
"What do you understand about the risk of transmission of HIV from woman to man, and man to woman?"
"Through intercourse, which body fluids are most likely to carry the virus?"
"What sexual activities do you consider to be 'risky'?"
"What is it that makes them 'risky'?"
"How many sexual partners have you had in the last year?"
"What do you know about the number of sexual partners and the risk of transmission of HIV?"

c) Protection of sexual partners

- Use condoms.
- Use spermicidal cream such as 'nonoxynol 9' which destroys HIV on contact
- Use a diaphragm (the 'cap')
- Avoidance of high-risk sexual activities such as unprotected penetrative intercourse (anal/rectal or vaginal).

"How might you protect your sexual partner?"
"What difficulties does this present in your relationship with him?"
"Have you thought about using condoms?"
"What might be the problems in using them?"
"How safe do you consider the condom to be?"
"Have you considered using spermicide cream as well as a condom?"
"Have you considered using a diaphragm or cap as well as your partner using a condom?"
"Do you think using the cap or diaphragm alone is sufficiently safe?"

Questions about the risks of kissing are a concern to all age groups, especially adolescents.

"What do you know about the risks of infection from kissing?"
"Is there anyway you can kiss without exchanging body fluids?"

People can be helped to consider less risky activities and to think about changing the emphasis of sex in their relationships.

"Have you ever thought of any other sexual activities that you and your partner might enjoy?"

d) Blood and blood products
HIV can be transmitted through infected blood. This can happen in various ways:
Blood transfusions

"How else can HIV be transmitted?"

Steps have been taken to safeguard the blood supply. Since October 1985 all blood donations have been screened for HIV in the UK. In the USA screening started in March 1985.

"Do you have any idea of what happens to blood that is donated?"

Blood supplies may not be screened in some countries.

"If you received donated blood in a foreign county do you think this could be any different?"

Blood should not be donated by those with HIV or who fall into any risk category such as:

- Homosexuals
- Bisexuals
- Haemophiliacs
- Intravenous drug users
- Those who have had sexual contact in African countries
- Prostitutes
- Sexual partners of all the above.

"Who do you consider should not donate blood?"
"Is the recipient likely to be at any risk from HIV from your blood?"
"Knowing that you are at risk for HIV do you know where you can get the HIV test?"
"Have you donated blood since 1979? Where and when?"
"Have you ever received a blood transfusion?"

Blood products:
such as factor VIII and IX, are used as replacement therapy by haemophiliacs. Prior to October 1985 the blood in UK and USA was not screened. Blood products are now screened and heat treated. (Blood cannot be heated).

"What do you understand about the safety of factors VIII and IX at the moment?"

"Do you know what is done to make the product safer?"

e) Other blood contamination risks:

- Sharing toothbrushes and razors

"What do you understand about the risks of sharing needles?"

"What do you understand about the risks associated with
- Tattooing
- Electrolysis
- Ear piercing
- Acupuncturing
- Sharing razors
- Sharing toothbrushes"

Intravenous drug users should be alerted to the risks associated with:

- Sharing needles
- Sharing equipment
- Sexual relationships
- Pregnancy

"Do you know how you might prevent getting or passing on HIV infection?"
"When you inject do you share needles?"
"What do you know about the risks to your sexual partners?"
"What can you do to reduce this risk?"
"Would you consider getting professional help for your drug problem?"
"Would you take part in a needle exchange scheme if it were available?"

f) Donation of semen, breast milk and organs

People at any risk should not donate:

- Blood
- Semen
- Untreated breast milk

Semen donation

A specimen is taken and stored, blood from the donor is taken at intervals to check for the HIV antibody before the semen is used. Organs being donated for transplant are tested for HIV.

"Do you donate semen?"
"Do you carry an organ donor card?"

"You mentioned that your child was conceived through artificial insemination by donor. Have you any concerns about HIV?"

g) Accidental exposure in health care settings

There are clinical and laboratory guidelines for handling HIV infected material and care of patients

- Needles should not be resheathed
- Use gloves and goggles where there is any risk
- Sharps should be carefully disposed of
- Use solvents or detergents (household bleach) where there has been blood or other body fluids spillage

Consult your infection control officer for further information. These guidelines may be used in the home when caring for patients with HIV infection.

"From your present knowledge, is there any specific risk in your work?"
"Are you likely to come into contact with patients body fluids?"
"Would this be through touching patients ("hands-on care") or working with samples in a laboratory?"
"What facilities do you have for disposal of needles and sharps?"
"Are you aware of local guidelines for infection control?"

"If you have a cut or open wound, or a skin problem on your hands, what procedure do you follow in relation to your work as a nurse?"
"If there is a spillage of Factor VIII or blood can you repeat to me the procedure you would follow?"
"What do you tell your teachers to do if you have a nose bleed?"

It is important to document the occupational transmission of HIV. Members of staff should be encouraged to participate in studies and surveillance projects.

"Would you be willing to enter a study of transmission to health care workers in relation to this incident?"
"If so, do you realize you might have your blood tested?"
"Might there be any other factors in your history that might affect the result?"

Decisions about pregnancy and procreation

h) Mother to infant
HIV transmission can take place during pregnancy from mother to fetus.

"Do you think there are risks of your baby being born with HIV infection?"
"Why have you chosen to think about having a child at this time?"

Woman who are at risk or HIV seropositive and who are considering pregnancy
There is insufficient knowledge now to pinpoint with accuracy the precise risk to both mother and the unborn child.
Discussion should include:

- The mother's chances of developing AIDS. This is thought to increase with pregnancy and, again with subsequent pregnancies
- Birth control measures
- Use of condoms, in addition to birth control measures

"If the obstetrician suggested that an HIV antibody test should be done on you, what would your view be?"

"What might be the risks to your own health if you were HIV positive and pregnant?"
"What do you know about the chances of developing AIDS through a second pregnancy?"
"How might you avoid pregnancy?"
"What, or who, would influence you the most in making a decision about having a child now?"

- Termination of pregnancy

"If you were pregnant now how might you view termination of the pregnancy if you were HIV antibody positive?"
"If you became ill who would care for your child or children?"
"If you were unwell and you had a child who had AIDS how might you cope?"

- Potential transmission of HIV to the child.

"What do you know about the chances of an infant developing AIDS from a mother who is infected with HIV?"

i) Women who are HIV seronegative whose sexual partner is HIV seropositive
This applies mainly to the wives and sexual partners of haemophiliacs, bisexual men and intravenous drug users.

Information should be given so decisions can be made with the maximum knowledge of potential risk. They might then be advised to reduce risk of transmission, where possible, by:

- Using condoms and birth control measures, preferably a diaphragm or cap, when not trying for a child.
- Limiting penetrative intercourse to the most fertile period.
- Observing HIV seropositive male partners absolute T_4 lymphocyte count. If it is declining he is likely to be more infectious.

"What do you know about the risks of a child being infected with the virus?"
"Who most wants a child: you, your husband, your family?"
"If you had a very sick child with HIV infection how might you cope?"
"If you had a child who subsequently died of AIDS, how might you cope with this?"
"If all of you in the family were seropositive how might you manage the uncertainty of developing AIDS?"
"What do you know about the risks of transmitting HIV if you do not use protective devices or birth control measures?"
"What do you know about the risks to your own health?"
"If you decide not to risk having a child what measures will you take to prevent this?"
"If you decide to go ahead and risk having a child who would help you if your husband died?"
"Who would look after the child if you developed AIDS and died?"

j) Breast feeding and HIV transmission

HIV virus has been detected in breast milk. There are, however, very few reports of this form of transmission since most children born to HIV seropositive mothers will already have been exposed to HIV. Information should be given about the pros and cons of breast feeding. The decision about recommending that a mother not breast feed a child should not be taken lightly, particularly where there are no breast milk substitutes, such as in parts of Africa.

"If there was uncertainty about breast milk would you consider another form of feeding?"
"What do you know about risks of transmission of HIV through breast milk?"
"What level of risk are you prepared to take?"

*HIV is **not** transmitted*
- Through sharing lavatories, bathrooms, kitchens
- By touching someone or breathing the same air as an infected person
- Kissing on the cheek or hugging
- Going to the same restaurant or pub or bar as an infected person
- Donating blood or having blood tests taken.

"What other ways do you think the virus might be transmitted?"
"Are there any ways that you are not sure about?"
"How is it **not** spread?"
"Do you think any of your friends would be concerned about social contact with you?"

II PERSONAL ISSUES

Fears of isolation and rejection

As a consequence of
- Social stigma
- Uncertainty
- Myths

Many people have to face the possibility of dealing with their illness alone.

"Who might you **want** to tell?"
"Who do you think you **ought** to tell?"
"How do you think she would react?"
"What worries you most about other people knowing?"
"What might be of help to you if he knew?"

"If you were rejected how might you handle the situation?"
"How might they show that they were rejecting you?"
"What is your greatest fear about being rejected?"
"What would help you the most in that situation?"
"How might you achieve this?"
"Now that you have more time to yourself, what are some of the things you are now able to do that you might not be doing if you were less isolated?"

Uncertainty
Uncertainty about:
- Whether AIDS will develop
- Whether friends and family will reject or support them
- Whether treatment might help
- The course of the illness.
- The lack of complete knowledge about HIV

"What is the most difficult aspect for you living with uncertainty?"
"What other aspects of your life are affected by uncertainty?"
"How have you coped with this in the past?"
"What are your views about managing these uncertainties?"
"You have just said that it is intolerable for you to sit back and let this illness destroy you. What would help you to feel you are doing the best you can, to take control of the situation?"
"If you knew you only had six months or a year to live how would you want to spend that time?"

Anxiety and stress
Symptoms of anxiety are often similar to those of HIV infection. Some of the more common sources of stress are:
- Family conflicts
- Problems with friends
- Problems at work
- Financial difficulties
- Housing problems

Identifying and addressing the anxiety and stress may be a step towards it's management.
Patients can be referred to their general practitioner, psychologist or psychiatrist for more specialized treatment.

"What is it that you do that makes you think you are anxious?"
"If your boyfriend were here, how would he describe your behaviour when you say you are anxious?"
"What is your main concern today?"
"Can you rank your concerns?"
"What is the worst aspect of this concern?"
"Who else knows you are concerned?"
"How might they know you are concerned?"
"If your friend were here today what might be his main concern about you?"
"Who might help you with this problem?
"Who or what might make it more difficult?"
"If you weren't concerned about your antibody test result, what else would you be worried about?"
"What were your main stresses before HIV and AIDS came onto the scene?"
"When you were stressed before what helped you the most?"
"When are you more stressed - in the morning or evening? When is it at its worst?"
"What else is happening to you around those times?"

Suicidal thoughts
The expression of suicidal thoughts should always be taken seriously and discussed with the patient.
Referral to a psychiatrist can be made if necessary.

"You say you feel helpless and hopeless and like giving up, have you ever thought about killing yourself?"

"How might you do it?"

AIDS/HIV issues that might
induce these ideas include:

- Knowledge of a fatal illness
- Constricted thinking under
  stress
- Not wanting to be a burden on
  others
- Fear of illness, pain and death
- Attempts to get attention
- Taking control of an
  illness that might take
  control of oneself

Insurance companies can refuse
to pay if they learn that
someone has commited suicide.

Religious and other beliefs

Some people have strong religious
or other beliefs which may
influence their views about:

- Sexuality and sexual behaviour
- Their illness and treatment
- Life-support measures
- Death
- Life after death
- Suicide
- The way they want to live
- Treatment

Body image

The visible effects of AIDS
can add to fears of identification,
stigma and rejection. These include:

- Extreme wasting
- Skin lesions, such as Kaposi's
  sarcoma

"Who else knows about your
plans?"
"How might they react if they
knew about this?"
"When have you thought about
killing yourself? Recently, or
only when you become very ill?"
"Now that you have told me,
what do you think I should be
doing about you?"

"Have you considered that if the
case gets to the coroner's court
your lover's name may be
implicated if the media get
involved?"

"Do you have any particular
religious beliefs?"
"You say your religion forbids
you to use condoms. How can
you protect yourself and your
sexual partner?"
"How do these beliefs fit with
your present condition?"
"How might these beliefs influence how you live with and cope
with your present condition?"
"Have there been dilemmas for
you in reconciling your religious
beliefs with your present
condition?"
"In what way are these views
similar or different to those of
your sexual partners or your
family?"

"What aspects of your condition
do you find most difficult to cope
with?"
"What might others find
difficult?"

Ways of coping physically and emotionally can be identified and explored. These include suggestions about:

- Cosmetic applications
- Clothing that disguises weight loss

"Are you more likely to be rejected by friends or by family or by colleagues?"

"Do you think they are more frightened of catching AIDS from you or being rejected themselves because of contact with you?"

"What are the ways you might find to cope with this?"

"What practical steps could you take to feel more confident in public?"

"Have you thought of using make-up?"

"Would you think of wearing loose clothes that disguise your being so thin?"

III RELATIONSHIP ISSUES

Sexual relationships

Effects of AIDS/HIV on both partners include:

- Fear of rejection
- Fear of infection
- Guilt and fear of disclosure of
  - promiscuity
  - infidelity
  - sexual preference
  - past sex history

"Have you discussed this with your sexual partner?"

"What might be his reaction?"

"How and when would you tell him, if at all you choose to discuss it with him?"

"If you had to confront someone with this information what are the words you would use?"

"What is the worst consequence that might happen if you were to tell them?"

"If you started using condoms now, would your wife be suspicious?"

"How would you deal with this?"

"What would help you tell your partner?"

"How might you tell previous sexual partners about your having HIV?"

"If you were able to tell your wife about your relationships with men, how do you think she would react?"

"If your partner decides to leave you, what would be the worst aspect, and how might you cope with it?"

Sexual partners
should have the opportunity to:
- Have the HIV antibody test
- Discuss concerns
- Be counselled with the patient where this is appropriate.

"Do you think your partner should have the HIV antibody test?"

"If they refuse what might be your advice?"

"What might be the benefits of coming for a discussion with your partner?"

"What might worry you most about doing this?"

"If your lover were here what might his reaction be to this conversation?"

The rights of individuals versus the public good is a common dilemma.

"We know you are HIV antibody positive and you insist you are not going to tell your wife. If you were in my position as counsellor and someone had just told you this what would be the dilemmas for you?"

Relationships in the family
Some possible consequences of having someone with AIDS/HIV in the family include:
- Less talk about AIDS for fear of worrying parents or child
- Less body contact.

"Do you talk less to your parents or brothers and sisters than you did before you knew you had HIV?"

"Do you notice any difference in the way your family treat you?"

Parents
Some parents may only know about their son's homosexuality or drug use at the time of illness and death.
It is stressful to keep secrets in the family.

"Do your parents know about your HIV status?"

"If you were to tell them how might they react?"

"Do you think your mother and father would react in the same way?"

Some parents may have chosen not to declare their knowledge about sexuality or drugs until highlighted by AIDS/HIV.

Parents reactions may include:
- Anger towards their child
- Guilt about their parenting
- Guilt about perhaps infecting their child
- Fear of stigma, isolation and rejection by friends, neighbours, colleagues
- Fears about the course of the illness
- Fears about the loss of their child
- Uncertainty about coping with death
- Fears for themselves of becoming infected.

"Do you think they would suspect anything at this point?"
"What might be the advantages or disadvantages of telling them?"
"Which of them might you choose to talk to first?"
"Do your parents know about your sexual activities?"
"What do you think would upset them more, telling them you are gay or that you have HIV?"
"If you choose not to tell any of your family and you became seriously ill and were admitted to an AIDS ward in this hospital how might this be handled?"
"What do you think are your parents greatest fears at this stage?"
"How might you help them?"
"What do your parents understand about AIDS?"
"How might you help them understand more?"
"How do you think your relationship with them might be different now they have this information?"
"How often do you talk to your parents about AIDS? Once a day, several times a day, every few days, never?"
"Do you think it might be easier for them to come and discuss this with you here, or would it be more difficult?"
"Do you think your sister would think you are protecting your parents more by talking, or not talking about AIDS and your concerns?"

Siblings

Some parents want to 'protect' other children from the information for fear of:

- Declaring the sexual preference of their son
- The effect on their other children
- The effect on other relationships at school, work and socially.

"Who else in the family would you think of telling?"

"Who would you find it easiest to tell?"

"What is it about them that makes it easier for you to talk to them?"

"How come it is easier to talk to your sister than it is to your brother?"

"If your neighbours were to find out because your younger brother told them, how might you deal with this?"

Children

Children of haemophiliacs, bisexual men and intravenous drug users have:

- Fears about death of the parent
- Fears for themselves of being infected with the virus
- Fears about reaction from friends.

"What do you think your children know about AIDS?"

"Knowing you have AIDS, what do you think is their greatest concern?"

"What do you think is the best way of telling them?"

"What would you advise them to say if they were asked about you at school?"

"Do you think they have stopped bringing friends home because of the fear of how they might react?"

"How might you help them to acquire information and confidence to mix with their friends?"

HIV positive child of HIV positive parent

"Does having a mother with HIV make it easier or more difficult for you?"

Relationships with friends

Fear of rejection can either lead people not to tell anyone, resulting in isolation, or lead to spreading the news in ways which may be regretted later

"Which of your friends would you want to tell?"

"How might this affect your relationship with them?"

The support and continuing relationship with friends can be of prime importance in helping the person to live with and cope with AIDS/HIV

Great care should be taken in choosing who to tell and at what stage they should be told

"How might you handle those friends who choose to turn their back on you?"

"So you have chosen not to tell anyone at this point about your HIV test. When do you think you would be ready to tell them?"

"You keep saying you feel lonely and isolated. If your best friend did know, do you think that might bring some relief to you?"

Relationship with employers and colleagues

There is no obligation to tell employers/colleagues.

There may be advantages and disadvantages to some people knowing.

Some implications include:

- Risk of dismissal
- Curtailed career prospects
- Adjustment of work routine
- Sick leave arrangements
- Stigma at work
- Reactions of colleagues and their families
- Pre-employment medicals
- Legal considerations.

With information and opportunities for rehearsal, people with HIV are likely to be more confident in how they might respond to unexpected questions. The result of any negotiations may be more successful.

"Who in the organization should be told, if at all anyone?"

"You have chosen not to tell your employers anything about your HIV status. If you start to take more days sick leave and they asked you to have a medical examination, have you thought how you would respond to them?"

"If you wanted to negotiate more suitable work conditions such as part-time employment, who might you talk to first and what would you say?"

"If you were dismissed what steps would you take?"

"Since your colleagues know you have haemophilia, and they may link it with AIDS, have you thought about what you would say to them if they asked about this?"

"If a colleague or your employer raised the issue of AIDS first and he asked you if you had AIDS - how would you handle it?"

"Is your relationship such that you might be able to negotiate more favourable conditions - such as part-time work?"

Relationships with school

There may be special concerns that children with AIDS/HIV and their parents may have to think about in their relationship with the school and other agencies.

There is no evidence that a child with HIV is any risk to others at school (or anywhere else) provided commonsense, precautions are taken.

Risk is different if children fight excessively or bite each other.

Children with HIV may be more vulnerable to common illnesses and infections. Normal developmental milestones may not be achieved and there may be learning difficulties.

Children who may have AIDS/HIV are:

- Haemophiliacs, infected by use of clotting factor VIII or IX before heat treatment killed the virus
- Children whose mothers are HIV seropositive and have passed on HIV during pregnancy
- Older children and adolescents who become infected by sharing needles (if they use drugs) or through sexual activities.

"Is there anyone at school who you think should know, such as headmaster, school doctor, or school nurse?"

"If your child had HIV what do you know about the possible effect of this on their development?"

"What signs of this might you look for?"

"How active is your child? Have you ever watched him play with other children? How does he behave with them?"

"As your child has haemophilia do you think they consider he is at risk for AIDS?"

"What would you say if you were asked?"

"If your son had a nose bleed at school what would you advise the teachers to do?"

"If you were teased at school about AIDS, how would you handle it?"

IV PRACTICAL ISSUES

Other agencies and professionals should be made accessible to those with AIDS/HIV, their families and those who care for them.

Referral procedures.

Well-planned referrals help towards co-ordinated care. Referrals should be negotiated with other professionals and agencies as far as is possible. This can help to clarify what cases are appropriate to refer and what can be reasonably expected from other professionals. Colleagues also need to understand what problems AIDS counsellors can help them with in their work setting. Since AIDS counsellors are a recent addition to paramedical services, referrals provide an opportunity to describe the tasks and role of the counsellor and to negotiate with the referrer if his or her expectations of the counsellor are different to what the counsellor can reasonably provide. Counselling can help the patient to see the potential benefit of referrals to specialists and at the same time help to reduce the patient's worries about a breach of confidentiality. Wherever possible, permission should be sought from the patient to discuss his case with colleagues or make a referral to another health care professional. If, through counselling, the message is conveyed to a patient that he stands to benefit from additional professional help and co-ordinated care, his refusal to concent to this is unlikely.

Social and community services
- Social workers
- Home helps
- Meals-on-wheels
- District nurses
- Volunteers, such as 'buddies' who befriend, support and help care for people with AIDS.

The needs of the individual should be carefully assessed, so that the help is appropriate. Patients should be encouraged to maintain control of their lives as far as possible.

Finances
Many people with AIDS are young and may not have accumulated sufficient savings to cope with illness. Parents who do not know that their child is ill (which is not uncommon) are obviously not in a position to provide financial support.

State benefits may need to be considered. There are also several private charities willing to provide financial help.

Some patients may lose their jobs. Others may be forced to give up work due to illness.

Loans and insurance (life and health) may be affected by a person's HIV status. People who are HIV antibody positive or who are thinking of having the test should be made aware of the potential constraints they may face.

Accommodation
The nature of a patient's accommodation is important to consider. This includes:

- Proximity to the hospital
- Physical conditions and facilities of the accommodation, for example, stairs and heating
- Whether the property is owned, rented, or council accommodation.
- Whether they are being harassed by neighbours.

Mobility

Mobility allowances and voluntary drivers may have to be considered. Proximity to the hospital and frequency of hospital visits must be planned for.

Legal and related issues

When the issue of Wills, Enduring Powers of Attorney, next-of-kin, and so on are discussed, there is an underpinning theme of the acknowledgement of the possibility of serious illness and death. It is preferable not to discuss these more sensitive issues in a first meeting with a patient unless he or she raises them.

Wills

Many young people have not considered making a will. The benefits of drawing up a will for those ill or those not yet ill should be stressed. Advice from a lawyer should be sought. Most hospitals can arrange for a will to be drawn up and witnessed.

Enduring Powers of Attorney

This can be a major source of practical help to those who are mentally well and who are able to make decisions, but physically unable to execute them.

Next-of-kin

If the next-of-kin is not identified then, after death, an immediate survivor will have to be traced and informed. Officially, information about a patient's health will only be discussed with an identified next-of-kin if the patient is too ill to give consent. The next-of-kin may be a family member, a lover or a close friend.

Guardianship of children

Provision will need to be made for the continued care of children whose parents are alive but perhaps in hospital, or who have abandoned their children.

Fostering and Adoption

Some children who have AIDS/HIV are put up for fostering and adoption because their natural parents may, in the view of a court, be unable to care for them. Prospective foster parents and parents who are adopting need to be aware of:

- The HIV status of the child
- Basic facts about AIDS
- Hygiene in the home
- Benefits and disadvantages of telling others the HIV status of the child
- The stigma they may face
- The impact of taking this child into the family where there may already be other children.

Court of Protection
If there are no relatives, and the patient is unable to make decisions or care for themselves, they can be made a ward of the Court of Protection. Social workers and lawyers can arrange this. Medical documentation of the patient's mental state and physical condition is required.

Acts of discrimination
Eviction and dismissal from work can occur and legal advice should always be sought. Sexual partners, friends, and the family of patients with HIV can also suffer. Acts of discrimination have been reported. The police and members of the health care team should always be informed of this.

Immigration visas and international mobility
Some countries require proof that a person is not infected with HIV. Authorities may demand that a person be tested for HIV at a port of entry. A person who refuses would not be permitted to enter the country. Those who are later found to have AIDS/HIV may be deported. If travel is contemplated, advice should always be sought on the latest position regarding AIDS/HIV in any particular country. Specialist advice should be sought about vaccinations for HIV antibody positive patients.

Public Health Acts
Many countries have acts for the control of infectious diseases. AIDS may be included as a notifiable disease. This would empower authorities to detain or isolate someone suspected of having HIV who is thought to be spreading it, or indeed someone who is already infected.

If in any doubt at all, people considering having the HIV antibody test or pursuing any decision that may result in their being restricted in some way should seek legal advice.

8
Pre-and post-HIV antibody test counselling interview

This chapter demonstrates how some of the ideas discussed in all previous chapters can be used in the context of pre- and post-HIV antibody test counselling.

The points that need to be covered are the same irrespective of whether the patient requests the test, or a doctor considers that the patient should have the test. It is important to convey to patients that the HIV antibody test is not a test for AIDS. HIV antibodies are a marker of infection. The detection of antibodies does not necessarily mean that the patient has AIDS or that they will develop AIDS. Giving bad news, such as a positive HIV antibody test result, is sometimes a difficult task. If patients are prepared for bad news through pre-test counselling, the task of giving a positive result is made much easier.

In counselling patients about having the HIV antibody test it is important to discuss current advantages and disadvantages to having this test. This helps patients to make informed decisions.

Some disadvantages

- Restrictions on mortgages and life insurance
- Possibility of increased stress and uncertainty
- Social stigma atttached to a positive HIV antibody result
- Stress from maintaining a secret
- Difficulties in making and maintaining relationships

Some advantages

- Knowledge of the result can reduce stress
- Decisions about the future might be made more easily
- Increased motivation to protect sexual partners.
- Symptoms can be identified and treated promptly
- Prophylactic treatment can be given.

This chapter is divided between the pre-and post-test counselling session.

CHECKLIST OF POINTS TO BE COVERED IN PRE-TEST COUNSELLING

1. Identify who you are in relation to the rest of the health care team
2. State how much time is available for counselling
3. Stress confidentiality

4. Ask what it is that has led to the patient coming for the test
5. Identify risk activities
6. Check knowledge about transmission and prevention
7. Discuss the 'window period' before HIV antibodies
   might develop
8. Discuss what the test is, and what it is not. It is not a test
   for AIDS
9. Identify whose idea it is that the person comes for the test
10. Assess why they are coming for the test at this stage
11. Discuss the personal implications of having the test and the
    meaning of the result, both negative and positive, for themself
    and others
12. Discuss the practical implications of the test such as life
    insurance, sexual relationships, work situations and medical
    follow-up
13. Describe the procedure for having blood taken, how long he will
    wait for the result and how he will be told about the result
14. Discuss healthy lifestyle irrespective of possible test result
    (safer sex, food, sleep, exercise, etc)
15. Identify how the patient will protect sexual partners in
    the interim
16. Discuss how the patient might cope with a negative or
    positive result
17. Discuss who the patient would *want* to tell and who the patient
    considers *ought* to be told
18. Identify what social support is available
19. Discuss the patient's views about the general practitioner
    sharing the patient's care with the hospital team if the HIV
    antibody test result is positive
20. Discuss who the patient can contact while waiting for the
    result, and the procedure for this
21. Arrange a follow-up interview.

ILLUSTRATIVE CASE
Mr Culbert, a 25 year old architect, telephoned his sexually transmitted diseases clinic for an appointment for a check up, including an HIV antibody test. He had attended the clinic on two previous occasions with gonorrhoea, which had been successfully treated. At that time he had one regular male sexual partner. He has been in a relationship with the same person for a few months. He recently told his parents that he is gay. He has one older married brother. He was interviewed by the AIDS counsellor before seeing the consultant. The following are excerpts from the interview.

Patient/counsellor conversation

Counsellor: "What is is that made you decide to come here today?"
Patient "I've come for my routine check up"

Counsellor: "In checking you today what are the most important things for us to know?"
Patient: "I'm feeling very anxious about my health"

Counsellor: "Can you tell me what it is about your health that is making you anxious?"
Patient: "I'm worried about AIDS"

Counsellor: "What is it about AIDS that worries you most?"
Patient: "Right now I'm worried that I might have caught it"
Counsellor: "How do you think you might have caught it?"
Patient: "Through somebody I met two months ago"
Counsellor: "How do you think you might have been infected?"
Patient: "Through having sex".
Counsellor: "What did you do whilst having sex that you think might have put you at risk?"
Patient: "I fucked this chap and I have been worried since"
Counsellor: "Do you do anything else apart from fucking?"
Patient: "Not really, but I know it is risky and I'm worried."

Explanation

Open-ended questions:
- Make no assumptions about why the person has come
- Allow the patient the first opportunity to define the problem as he sees it **without** the counsellor defining it as a problem.

Using his words, the counsellor begins to get the patient to define his concern in relation to the purpose of the clinic visit that day. This acknowledges that the definition of the problem may change over time.

The patient has defined his major worry. The counsellor is still not making any assumptions about the nature of the worry, or the potential impact of AIDS on the patient.

The patient is helped to rank his major concern.

Identify what the patient considers to have been a risk.

The counsellor begins to:
- Check knowledge
- Identify risk activity

'Sex' means different things to different people. A statement about sexual activities is needed in order to clarify the risk.

More precise information about activities is explored.
Using the patient's words helps to keep the interview neutral.
Acceptance of their terminology is conveyed.

Counsellor: "What have you in mind to do about this worry?"
Patient: "I don't really know - perhaps I should have the AIDS test"
Counsellor: "Can you tell me what you know about this test?"
Patient: "The test will tell me if I've got AIDS"
Counsellor: "No, the test will not tell whether you have AIDS right now. It will only tell whether you have come into contact with the virus in the past. It will not tell whether or not you have AIDS. So if this result is positive, from what you've heard can you clarify for me what this means?"
Patient: "Oh, so it just tells me that I've been infected in the past. What are my chances of getting AIDS?"
Counsellor: "From what you have heard from the media or elsewhere what do you understand about your chances of getting AIDS?"
Patient: "I don't know. I've heard 30 per cent and one doctor said 100 per cent will get AIDS?"
Counsellor: "Well there are differing views about this at the moment. At present we cannot be certain about how many will ultimately develop AIDS. Much is still unknown".
Patient: "Does that mean that if I was positive I could infect others?"
Counsellor: "Yes, if your HIV antibody result is confirmed to be positive it is presumed that you will remain infected and infectious for life. If it is positive who would you want to tell?"
Patient: "Um....well maybe just my present partner".

Encourage the patient to focus on something he can do about the worry. Let the suggestion for the test come from the patient if possible.
Knowledge about the test is checked.

The counsellor checks what is known:
- Misinformation is corrected
- Short explanations are given
- Information is checked by first getting the patient to repeat in his words what he has understood before more information is provided

Again, first:
- Assess the patient's knowledge
- Source of information

If the counsellor is up to date with current studies he will have more confidence in responding to what patients ask and in addressing uncertainty.

Information is given. This leads to discussion about how AIDS issues affect other people.
The use of hypothetical questions helps the counsellor to explore, with the patient, some of the implications of having HIV.

Counsellor: "What would be your hesitation in telling him?"

Patient: "I don't know what would happen to our relationship".

Counsellor: "If you were to tell him what do you think might be his greatest concern?"

Patient: "That he too might have caught it".

Counsellor: "Right, so if you decided to tell him how might you begin to talk to him about this?"

Patient: "I wouldn't know how to start".

Counsellor: "Let's try and rehearse the words you might use right now".

Patient: "I could say I went for my check up and I'm worried about AIDS. It affects us both so could you come with me next time to the clinic?"

Counsellor: "Yes, I've heard from you that you would find ways of making a start in telling him about your worries. And what if your HIV antibody test result turned out to be negative?"

Patient: "That would mean I would be alright".

Counsellor: "Alright in what way?"

Patient: "That I haven't got AIDS".

Counsellor: "From what we know that may not be correct. It is possible to be infected and not show antibodies for several weeks or more".

Patient: "So that means I may be infected and I won't know for a while?"

Counsellor: "It is important for us to establish when you think you might have been infected first".

Patient: "I don't know. Maybe my present lover or anyone else over the last 2 years".

Develop the relationship theme.
Address the anxiety.

This addresses:
- The relationship.
- Some of the possible different views of the relationship.

If situations are thought about in advance it is possible that they might be better managed.

Acting out the hypothetical situation helps the patient rehearse the most feared aspect.
This can help reduce some of the anxiety.

The patient's own resources are identified and reinforced.
The implications of a positive and negative result are explored.

The patient's view is challenged.
Because of the 'window period' it may not be possible to reassure all patients.

Discuss uncertainty in relation to the 'window' period in which the patient may be infected, but antibodies may not be detectable.

Counsellor: "If the result is negative that means we cannot be sure you are not infected or infectious. Whilst you don't know for certain, how might you protect your sexual partner and yourself if you are going to have penetrative intercourse?"

Patient: "I suppose condoms".

Counsellor: "Are there any other things you think might be affected by your having the test done?"

Patient: "Well I know there is a problem with insurance. But would I have to tell my boss?"

Counsellor: "Well, can you think of any advantages and disadvantages of him knowing?"

Patient: "I can't think of any advantages offhand, but it might affect my career prospects and he may tell others. So it might not be a good idea to tell him".

Counsellor: "Is there anything else you would like to say or ask that you haven't had a chance to ask so far?"

Patient: "Nothing to ask, but I'm not 100 per cent sure about having the test. What do you recommend?"

Counsellor: "From what I've seen and heard today, I get the impression that you have already thought about a number of the issues that go with having the test. Given a little more time I have the impression that you will come to the right decision yourself. This decision doesn't have to be made now. I would like to see you in a week to discuss this further. Perhaps you might like to think more, between now and that time, about some of the things we spoke about today. Would you like to discuss some of these issues now with the consultant?"

Personal and public health issues are considered:
- High risk group
- High risk activities
- Safer sex practices
- Prevention of transmission.

The patient is helped to think about other practical implications.

This helps the patient to make a more informed decision.

In the context of a structured interview this gives the patient a chance to ask questions or raise any further issues not already discussed.

The aim is to put the decision-making back to the patient. His ability to do so is assessed and positively connoted. This helps to reinforce his confidence in making decisions. The counsellor need not then be left with the patient's dilemma.

Between having the test and receiving the results, patients can become very anxious. The patient should be told who he can contact if he becomes very anxious.

POST-TEST COUNSELLING INTERVIEW

The post-test counselling interview, although separate to the pre-test counselling interview, is inextricably bound to it. That is, how the HIV antibody test result is given, and how the patient will cope with the news depends on how he has been prepared for a possible positive result through pre-counselling. Test results should never be given unless there is sufficient time to allow the patient to discuss his concerns. It is not uncommon for patients to feel suicidal especially if there is no opportunity to talk about the meaning and implications of the result for him. It is preferable to give results at the beginning of a week when more staff may be available to offer support and further information over the following days.

It should always be remembered that no matter how many positive HIV antibody test results a doctor has given, almost every patient experiences shock and distress. Patients are often unable to absorb any information after they have heard the result. Aspects of the post-test counselling session may have to be repeated from time to time. The approach that has been outlined in this book is of particular use when patients are in shock. Through the method of asking questions the patient becomes active and is re-engaged after the shock. This, in turn, prevents patients from simply 'switching off' whilst the counsellor goes into long explanations.

CHECKLIST OF POINTS TO BE COVERED
IN POST-TEST COUNSELLING

1. Give the result
2. Check what the patient understands by the result
3. If negative: suggest retest in three months, if appropriate.
Reinforce strategies for prevention of transmission and safer sex
4. If positive:
Identify immediate concerns:
Discuss who the patient might tell about the result
Dicuss what the patient might tell others
Discuss when the patient might tell others
Discuss how the patient might tell others and role play this
   with him
Discuss how the patient plans to spend next few hours and days
Identify what difficulties the patient foresees and how he might
   deal with them
Help the patient to identify who else he might turn to for support
Encourage the patient to ask questions
Discuss health maintaining behaviours such as safer sex, good
   diet, sleep, exercise etc
Assure the patient that the reaction of shock, anger or disbelief is
   quite common

> Discuss medical follow-up procedures (including shared care
>   with general practitioner) and benefit of prompt identification
>   and treatment of symptoms
> Give information about local support organizations
> Always offer a follow-up appointment.

Mr Culbert returned a week later. He decided to have the HIV antibody test and told his sexual partner about the previous visit to the sexually transmitted diseases clinic. His result was HIV antibody positive.

Patient-counsellor conversation

Counsellor: "It is a week since I saw you last when we took a blood sample. What is the result that you are expecting?"
Patient: "Well, I always expect the worst, so I guess it is positive"

Counsellor: "The result we have is positive. What does that mean to you?"
Patient: "Oh no!...I'm going to get AIDS?"

Counsellor: "What do you remember from the last interview about the meaning of this result?"
Patient: "OK - I know it doesn't mean that I've got AIDS but I'm so afraid."
Counsellor: "What are you most afraid of."
Patient: "Dying..."
Counsellor: "What is it about dying that you fear most?"
Patient: "I'll be alone - it'll be a slow, painful death and people with AIDS look so dreadful. Everyone would know I'd have it."

Explanation

Breaking bad news is difficult. The purpose of the interview is immediately defined. An opportunity is found in the first few minutes to give the news so that the rest of the session can be used to help the patient deal with this.
Check that the patient understands the meaning of a positive result. His reply indicates that he may not have fully understood the meaning of the antibody test result.
His knowledge is checked. The patient's concerns are identified and addressed. The counsellor does not impose his own views or give long explanations.
Concerns are identified and ranked.

Use the patient's words. This helps the counsellor to keep pace with the intensity of the patient's feelings. 'Dreaded issues' about dying are inextricably a part of AIDS. Opportunities must be found to talk about them.

Counsellor: "Of all of these which is the worst aspect for you?"
Patient: "Being alone I guess."

The main concern of the patient is addressed. Not all of his concerns can be adequately addressed at one time.

Counsellor: "If you had a choice, who would you want to be with you? And how might you let them know?"
Patient: "I'd like my parents, my mother to be around with me. But they don't even know I'm gay."
Counsellor: "If you told them this result how might they react?"
Patient: "They'd be really upset."

The idea that there are some ways that the patient can be in control of his situation is introduced.

The patient is helped to think about his relationships with others who are important to him. The counsellor focuses on behaviour.

Counsellor: "Which of your parents would be more upset, and how might they show it?"
Patient: "My mother would be upset about AIDS - uh - I mean the antibody test result. She'd cry a lot. My father - I can't say, he'd be angry about my being gay."
Counsellor: "How might he show he was angry?"
Patient: He wouldn't say it, but he just wouldn't talk to me for a while. So I can't tell him you see."
Counsellor: "Do you think they would be more upset and angry if they found out at a later stage - say if you were ill - or if you told them now?"
Patient: "...that's a good question..."
Counsellor: "At this stage who do you think needs to know this result? What about your general practitioner?"
Patient: "I don't often see him anyway."
Counsellor: "Why do you think I mention your general practitioner?"
Patient: "Because he might have to treat me if I was ill, but not so ill that I'd have to be in hospital. How would I know if I was getting AIDS?"

This is a 'difference' question which gives information about relationships in the family and who might be available to help the patient. Again the focus is on behaviour.

The counsellor focuses on specific behaviour. He makes the patient describe in concrete terms statements about emotional conditions.
Challenging the patient's views helps him to view the problems differently.

General practitioners are an essential part of the medical team and patients should be encouraged to see them for early identification and, if possible, treatment of symptoms.
Re-emphasize the advantages of the general practitioner knowing the result. Stress that the result would not be passed on to the general practitioner without the patient's consent.

Counsellor: "From what you know, what might be some symptoms?"

Knowledge about AIDS is checked.

Patient: "Losing weight, skin rashes, colds that won't go away."

Counsellor: "Having heard that you are HIV antibody positive, what are you going to do immediately after leaving the clinic?"

Get a detailed description of how the patient intends to spend the next few hours, days etc. This forms part of the assessment of how he may cope with the news.

Patient: "Well, I've got to meet my boss for lunch, and now I just can't face it."

Counsellor: "If you don't want to face him how will you handle this?"

Help the patient to manage his situation in a practical way.

Patient: "I'll phone him and tell him I'm ill - and I'm going home."

Counsellor: "Do you think you'd be better at home on your own or making the effort through lunch?"

This is a challenging question which may open up other ideas and options.

Patient: "I suppose I should try to manage lunch with him. But keeping secrets like this is so hard."

Counsellor: "Yes it can be. It might help you to get in touch with an organisation called 'Body Positive' who will arrange for you to meet with other people in a similar situation. With these people you can share the secret. But maybe you need to think about who else to tell and how to tell them, before we meet again."

Social support and community resources should be made available to the patient.
Not all issues can be dealt with in a single session.

Patient: "...yeah. What about my partner though? Maybe he's also got it, or maybe I got it from him."

Counsellor: "Have you thought more about how you might tell him?"

Focus on behaviour.

Patient: "He wants to know my result straight away - so it won't be too difficult."

Counsellor: "What do you imagine will be his immediate reaction?"

Help the patient think about the reaction of others.

Patient: "Oh, he panics."

Counsellor: "When he panics what do you normally do?"
Patient: "Leave him alone for a while."
Counsellor: "What do you think will be his greatest concern?"
Patient: "That he has got it from me."
Counsellor: "Have you any ideas about how you might handle that?"
Patient: "I just can't say right now. He needs to have the test too. Perhaps you could see us together."
Counsellor: "Fine, I would like to see you next week on Tuesday and I would be happy to see your partner with you. Meanwhile, if you have any concerns, you can contact me here in office hours, but should I not be available you can speak to Dr Johnson or Sister Yales."

Draw out normal coping responses.

The partner may have a different concern to that of the patient.

The focus here is practical. The patient's responsibility for finding solutions is encouraged.

Knowledge about a follow-up appointment helps to contain some anxiety. A procedure is outlined for how the patient can be in touch with the counsellor between sessions should he feel acutely distressed. This keeps in mind the possibility of suicidal thoughts. The counsellor only offers what he can realistically fulfil.

9
Cases to illustrate approaches and techniques of counselling

Twenty-two cases are described and the theory behind the counselling approach is outlined in each. Each case provides insight into a situation which was dealt with in a clinical setting. The aim of this chapter is to describe some of the difficulties for the patient and the counsellor and to present a procedure for dealing with them. It should be remembered that although some situations appear similar, in reality each case is different. It is for the reader to use what applies in his or her work setting. Throughout this work names and details have been altered so as to protect the confidential nature of clinical material.

CASE A   HAVING CHILDREN WHERE ONE OF THE PARTNERS IS HIV ANTIBODY POSITIVE

Description of the problem
Mr Steven Peyton (32), unmarried, has been known to be HIV antibody positive for 18 months. He became infected through sexual contact with another man. His female sexual partner, Jean, is, to date, HIV seronegative. They want a child. Mr Peyton's medical surveillance is from the general practitioner and he has referred them to the counsellor.

Stage of HIV infection:
HIV antibody positive; no clinical symptoms
T_4 cells dropping over the last 2 months
Girlfriend HIV antibody negative, to date

Individual's stage in life
Adult. Peak of working life

The individual in relation to the stage of the family's development
Left home, cohabiting, unmarried, thinking about having children and getting married.

Principal issues to be addressed

- HIV infection risk to female partner
- Risk of HIV to female partner
- Risk of HIV to unborn child
- Effect on relationships if:
    - they have a child
    - the mother becomes infected, unwell or dies
    - the father becomes unwell or dies
    - the child becomes unwell or dies
    - they choose not to have children.

- Other ways of having children, for example, artificial insemination by donor

- Staff dilemma: problem of not advising but giving information, even when it may be limited and inconclusive.

How to address these issues

Question 1 Dr Kay asked me to see you today. What do you think he had in mind for us to be talking about?

Question 2 What, precautions are you taking to prevent pregnancy if any at all?

Question 3 How come you've thought about having children now? What would be the view of each of your parents if they were in the room now?

Question 4 If you decided not to risk the possibility of infecting the mother and child, and thus never have a baby, how do you see your future together? Are there any reasons, apart from HIV, that might influence the decision about having children?

Question 5 Have you thought about other ways of having children, such as artificial insemination by donor?

Question 6 If you decided to take the risk and go ahead and have a child, and your boyfriend died, have you thought about how you might cope? And if Jean became infected and ill who might care for the baby? How might it affect your relationship if you had to care for a baby who was very unwell?

CASE B MEDICAL SURVEILLANCE: ADDRESSING 'DREADED' ISSUES

Description of the problem

Mr Davids (29) is a homosexual man who is HIV antibody positive, and has been under medical surveillance in the department of genitourinary medicine for the past year. He was referred to the AIDS counsellor by a consultant in that clinic who was concerned that the patient was reporting feeling tired and had lost weight. Furthermore he had lymphadenopathy and his T_4 cell count had dropped consistently over the last three months. The consultant said that he was finding it difficult to manage this patient and to talk to Mr Davids. In the past, the patient had written complaining that he thought that important information was being kept from him by the medical team. When the consultant tried subsequently to discuss some issues with Mr Davids, he became dismissive, folded his arms and indicated that he was coping well.

Stage of HIV infection
HIV antibody positive, lymphadenopathy, low T_4 count, weight loss. Some clinical signs of illness becoming evident

Individual's stage in life
Adult: left home only 18 months ago. No ambivalence about his
sexuality. Trying to establish a career

The individual in relation to the stage of the family's development
Only child. Close contact with mother. Father died 5 years ago
Relationship with an older man

Principal issues to be addressed
 • **Paradox: "Tell me everything doctor, but only give me good news."**
   This theme, which can be expressed in many different ways, is
   common where there is uncertainty and anxiety
 • What to tell patients about their illness and when to tell them
 • Talking about 'dreaded issues' (ventilation, resuscitation, irreversible
   illness, neurological impairment, death and dying) while patients are
   not too ill to prevent them from making their views known about how
   they might wish to be cared for
 • How the patient and others can be more involved in the patient's care
 • Helping staff deal with the above issues in order to enhance patient
 care and reduce staff stress

How to address these issues
The following are guidelines and questions that may be used to address some
of these issues:

(1) A general principle to be applied when patients put members of the health
care team in a difficult position regarding their care is to show the patient that
what they are asking for cannot realistically be given.

 • *How will we know from you exactly what you want to know about your
   illness? And how will you indicate it?*
 • *What sort of things do you want to be told about? And when do you want
   to be told about them? Is there anything you do not want to be told
   about?*
 • *If you were in my situation, what would you be advising the patient?*

(2) While patients are relatively well, 'dreaded issues' can be most effectively addressed. These issues are still hypothetical and the patient has some
distance from the critical events.

 • *If you became so ill that you needed to be resuscitated or ventilated,
   what are your views about this now?*
 • *If you were unable to make decisions for yourself, who would you want
   to make them for you?*

(3) Indirect questions can be less confronting. In trying to engage the support
of relatives, it is possible to ask:

- *What do you think would be the effect on your relationship with your boyfriend if your mother were to spend more time with you down here in London?*

Identify those people who are close to the patient. It should not always be presumed that family members are emotionally closer to the patient than, for instance, friends.

- *Between your boyfriend and your mother, and perhaps anyone else, who would you name as your 'next-of-kin?' Who else would you like to be kept informed about your illness?*

(4) It should not be assumed that being more open with patients solves all management problems. One might ask of a colleague who is concerned about a patient:

- *If you were able to be more open with the patient about his deteriorating medical condition, would it make it easier or more difficult to manage him? In what way?*

CASE C   A ROUTINE MEDICAL EXAMINATION: TALKING ABOUT AIDS/HIV

Description of the problem
Miss Burns (48) has consulted her general practitioner three times over the last four months. She has been complaining of fatigue, itchiness, some weight loss and more recently, bruising. Despite careful examination and tests the general practitioner attributed these to middle-age depression. He was concerned, however, about the patient's platelet count. The general practitioner noted that the patient had had a blood transfusion in 1983. He wanted to do an HIV antibody test, but he was not sure about how to introduce the subject with this patient.

Stage of HIV infection
Possible symptoms of HIV infection
Not yet been tested for HIV

Individual's stage of life
Adult, no previous sexual partners
Single, menopausal, works as public relations officer
Lives alone

The individual in relation to the stage of the family's development
Some contact with younger married sister
Parents died six years ago. No other relatives

Principal issues to be addressed
- How best to broach the possibility of HIV in the context of a routine medical examination
- Identify potential risks of HIV
- Assess how the patient might cope, and who else there is around her to provide support if the HIV antibody test proves to be positive

How to address these issues
The general practitioner:
(1) States that he is concerned about her many symptoms and that he has not yet come up with a satisfactory explanation for them
(2) Asks the patient if she has any idea about what is causing the symptoms. Enquires about what the patient may know about risks of infection from blood transfusions. He asks her if she has thought about AIDS
(3) Asks the patient if she thinks she might have had any other risk for HIV (drugs, sex)
(4) States that he would like to do an HIV antibody test. He explains the procedure and the meaning of the result. He explores how she might cope if the result were positive, and what he would offer her in the way of care, management and support. (see Chapter 8 for pre-and post-test counselling procedure)
(5) Explores who else is available to support her if she might need it. Next-of-kin are identified
(6) Offers a follow-up appointment and clarifies the times he is available in the interim to answer any questions or help her with any worries. He asks patient how she will spend the next hours and days until the next appointment, when she will receive the result of the HIV antibody test.

CASE D   A BLOOD DONOR WHO IS FOUND TO BE HIV ANTIBODY POSITIVE

Description of the problem
Miss Flagstaff (32), who works at the Foreign Office, has recently returned from Africa where she was posted for the previous 18 months. Before she went overseas she had always been a regular blood donor and she resumed donating blood on her return. HIV antibodies were detected in this first donation. It was subsequently revealed that she had had one sexual contact

in Africa. She was now contemplating the resumption of a relationship with a married man she had known for 5 years before going to Africa. He had divorced a month before her return. She was referred to the consultant at the Blood Transusion Centre for counselling:

Stage of HIV infection:
HIV antibody positive. Second sample sent for confirmatory testing

Individual's stage of life:
Single adult. Foreign service career. Independent
Has had two previous sexual relationships

The individual in relation to the stage of the family's development:
Been in a relationship with a married man for 5 years. Considering marrying him. He has recently divorced. Limited contact with her own parents.

Principal issures to be addressed
- Test stored samples of previous donations from donor (if available) to identify when she might have seroconverted
- Trace recipients of previous blood donations to identify when she may have seroconverted and to prevent further transmission
- Break bad news to an unsuspecting donor
- Discuss knowledge about AIDS/HIV and the meaning of the HIV antibody test result
- Discuss who the donor might want to tell, who she thinks should be told, and when they should be told
- Identify true risk for epidemiological purposes
- Consider, with the donor, whether to inform and screen her sexual partner, his ex-wife and possibly his children
- Assess the reactions of the donor. Consider with her how she will spend the next few days or so and how she might cope
- Arrange for referral for medical surveillance and further counselling.

Procedure for Screening Donations

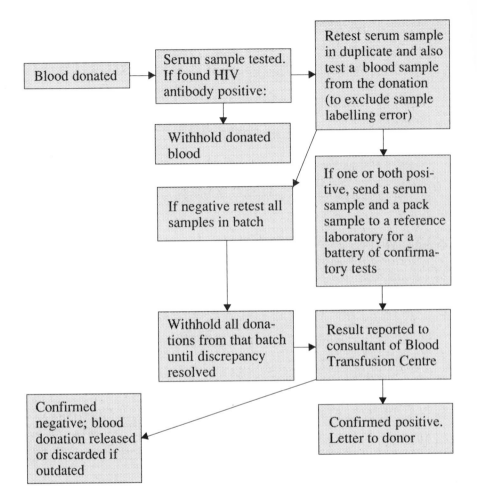

Framework for addressing the issues

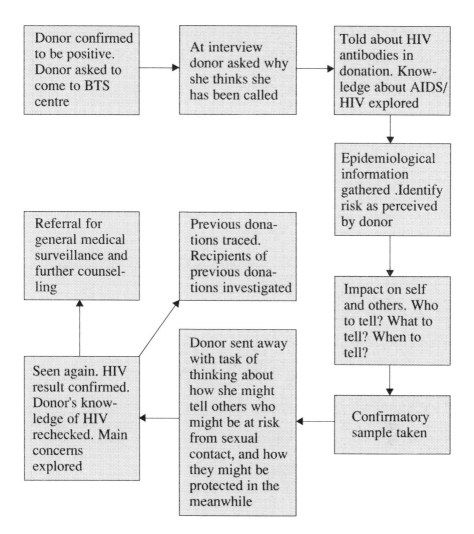

Acknowledgement The advice of Dr Patricia Hewitt and her colleages at the North London Blood Transfusion Centre is gratefully acknowledged.

CASE E INTRAVENOUS DRUG USERS AND AIDS/HIV

Description of the problem
The ward sister in a medical unit contacted the AIDS counsellor after a young woman, (19), had been admitted with hepatitis. From the patient's history it was presumed that she was infected after sharing needles with other intravenous drug users. The ward sister considered that an HIV antibody test should be carried out, and the consultant in charge agreed with this. None of the ward staff were themselves worried about being infected with HIV as full hepatitis precautions were already being taken with this patient and on the ward generally.

Stage of HIV infection
At risk - but not yet tested

Individual's stage of life
Single. Unemployed. In late teens

The individual in relation to the stage of the family's development
Left the family home at age 15
No contact with parents
In daily telephone contact with older sister

Principal issues to be addressed
- Unstable and 'chaotic' individual and family background
- Patient may be unlikely to take advice or to attend for follow-up appointments
- Health eduction in relation to drug use and general hygiene
- Reduction of risk activities (needle exchange, safer sex, birth control)
- Referral to drug dependency unit and drug outreach organization

How to address these issues
(1) Introduce yourself and clearly state the confidential nature of the interview

(2) Identify and use the specific words the patient uses in relation to her drug use and sexual activites

(3) Elicit the patient's main concerns. Then ask where AIDS ranks as a concern. Assess knowledge about transmission of HIV and prevention. Give information

(4) Discuss living conditions, social support, daily activities, and what she would do if she became ill. Be practical and concrete.
Identify who she might turn to if she would want further help

(5) Discuss all aspects of the HIV antibody test. If she declines to have the test, discuss what she would do to prevent transmission of HIV or becoming infected (if she is not already infected). Outline potential risks to children and to herself if she were to become pregnant and was infected with HIV.

(6) Offer a further appointment. Arrange for her to meet an outreach worker with specialist knowledge about drug use. Refer her to other agencies if this is appropriate, such as social services.

CASE F COUNSELLING IN RELATION TO ANTIVIRAL TREATMENT

Background
There is an increasing range of antiviral drugs available for patients who have HIV infection and AIDS. None are, as yet, a complete cure. These drugs are being used at different stages of illness.

Issues to be discussed with the patient

- Define whether this is a drug trial or a established drug. This will influence the definition of the purpose of giving the drug and the patient's likely response. Some patients are more inclined to enter a drug trial in the service of science, while they may be less certain about exposing themselves to potent drugs which have severe side effects, but are well-established in treatment.
- Consider what definition of illness is being given when antiviral drug therapy is offered and and the implications of this. For example, "This is a last resort"; "This is a known successful treatment for your infection"; "We are using this drug prophylactically".
- It is important to discuss practical issues.
  Assess the ability of the patient to attend for regular monitoring at the hospital or health centre. Consider whether patients are able to wake themselves during the night (if this is necessary) in order to take their medication; or whether the drug would impair their mobility.
- Clarify that antiviral drugs are a treatment, not a cure. Mention the possible side-effects and indications for withdrawal of treatment. Discuss with patients how they might view things if this treatment is not successful, or if the drug has to be stopped.

Issues the health care team might consider in offering drug treatment
(1) Are there the financial resources to supply the drug over a potentially long period of time?

(2) Is this a drug trial or routine treatment?

(3) How might they respond to patients who ask for the drug in a clinic where it is not available?

(4) Do they have the resources for the regular and detailed monitoring of these patients?

(5) What problems might arise where patients live longer but there is still uncertainty about their condition?

(6) How might members of staff respond to patients' interest in 'alternative therapy'?

(7) Is it safe, in the consultant's opinion, to give this patient large supplies of a drug to take home?

(8) How can members of the health care team present a case within their district for extra funds to pay for such drug treatment?

(9) Consider how and when to discuss difficult issues with patients, such as stopping the treatment because of side-effects.

Summary

It is important to counsel patients before antiviral treatment is offered. If the most feared aspects are considered at an early and appropriate stage, patients may be better prepared if changes in their clinical care have to be made. Unrealistic expectations of treatment may arise less frequently.

CASE G ADOLESCENT WITH HIV: ENTERING INTO RELATIONSHIPS

Description of the problem

Steven, aged 17, has severe haemophilia and he is HIV antibody positive. He is studying for his A-levels and he attends the Haemophilia Centre every 6 months for a review of his health. Steven is on a home-treatment regime which has helped him to be independent at an early age. At his last review session he stated. "I think I've found a girlfriend at last!"

Stage of HIV infection:
HIV antibody positive and asymptomatic

Individual stage of life:
Preparing to leave school; achieving independence; beginning to form significant relationships

The individual in relation to the stage of the family's development:
Second child preparing to leave home
Parents facing the 'empty nest'

Principal issues to be addressed
- Clarification of activities associated with the risk of transmission of HIV (e.g. intercourse, kissing)
- Knowledge about prevention of pregnancy and transmission of HIV and in this case, inheritance of haemophilia
- Explain how young people form and maintain relationships in the context of HIV
- Explain the impact of this new relationship on patient, his parents and others

How to address these issues
The following are excerpts from an interview:

Steven: I think I've found a girlfriend at last!

Counsellor: OK, what does she know about you, in relation to AIDS and haemophilia?

Steven: I've told her nothing ...I'm worried my one and only chance will pass me by!

Counsellor: At what point in any potential sexual relationship might you be able to talk to someone about this?

Steven: When I know the girl really likes me.

Counsellor: What are your main concerns?

Steven: Well, what about kissing? D'you think it's safe?

Counsellor: As we've discussed before, the main known risk from kissing is if there is any exchange of blood. It's unlikely that HIV is passed on through saliva alone. However, if people want to eliminate every possible risk, deep kissing should be avoided. If you were to have sexual intercourse, how would you talk about condoms and protection?

Steven: I don't really know....

Counsellor: How much have you talked about AIDS with your friends at school?

Steven: They know I've got haemophilia. None of them would ever think of using condoms anyway.

Counsellor: Have you ever thought that other people might also be at risk, and that the advice these days is for everyone to take precautions, such as using condoms. Birth control pills are not good enough. Maybe your girlfriend would think that you were caring if you insisted on condoms.

Steven: But who would want me when there are problems about my having children - I mean the haemophilia and the AIDS thing? This is what my mother worries about.

Counsellor: There are many people who can't have children for lots of reasons. Some never find a partner; some have medical problems; and some choose not to have children. So if you find ways of talking to this girl maybe she will see things differently. She might like you for other reasons.

Steven: Maybe when I get to know her better it will be easier to talk about this....

Counsellor: Yes, in my experience of counselling many young men in your position, they seem to find girls and find ways of telling them. They also seem to find the right time and the right place to do this as well.

Later on in the same session

Counsellor: What would happen if this relationship didn't work out?
Steven: I think my parents would be more upset than I would. Secretly they think I have no chance of getting married anyway.
Counsellor: What ideas have you now got for talking to them about it?
Steven: Maybe I'll talk to my brother first.
Counsellor: From what I've heard today Steven, you do have some particular problems because of your haemophilia and HIV. These have to be taken into consideration, as you have been doing, whenever you enter into relationships. However, all people of your age, whether they are HIV antibody positive or negative, have to think about using condoms and protecting each other from the risks of infection - both men and women. Making and keeping relationships is not easy for anyone. You've managed haemophilia over these years and you have attained a great deal of independence - and this experience should help you deal with this additional problem now and in the future.

CASE H SELF DISCLOSURE: THE MANAGEMENT OF ACUTE DISTRESS

Description of the problem

Mr McLoughlin (63), a business manager, was visiting the UK from the USA. He came to an outpatient clinic where he was investigated and treated for persistent diarrhoea and an allergic skin condition. The senior registrar considered that Mr McLoughlin might be at risk for HIV. The patient consented to an HIV antibody test after eventually declaring his homosexuality. The test proved to be positive. In spite of all previous efforts to prepare Mr McLoughlin for the result through counselling, he was shocked and devastated on receiving the news. He subsequently made many unscheduled visits to the senior registrar, telephoned him several times each week, and he wept throughout most sessions. Mr McLoughlin was very worried that the identification of AIDS, perhaps on his death certificate, would unmask his homosexuality which he maintained he had managed to keep secret from his family. The senior registrar was concerned about Mr McLoughlin's ability to cope and he thought that he might be suicidal. The patient was referred to an AIDS counsellor.

Stage of HIV infection:
HIV antibody positive. p24 antigen positive
Evidence of symptoms of AIDS

Individual stage of life:
Mature adult. Reaching retirement. Single. Living alone

The individual in relation to the stage of the family's development:
Older brother recently widowed. Looks to the patient for comfort in his bereavement. Both have had to face illness and death in the family. The patient described his brother as being 'close' but they never discussed his homosexuality

Principal issues to be addressed
- Suicide risk
- How to use counselling time efficiently and effectively in a busy clinic
- Strategies for sharing the responsibility for the psychosocial care of the patient in order to relieve some pressure on medical staff
- Who else the patient wants to be involved in his care, and to link him with other relevant community support
- Opportunities for the patient to talk about his homosexuality and the implications of AIDS/HIV for him

Summary of how the case was managed
The patient was seen three times at weekly intervals with the AIDS counsellor and the senior registrar, before he returned to the United States.

Session 1
(1) Knowledge about HIV and AIDS was explored
(2) The patient was helped to talk about homosexuality and his relationship with his brother
(3) The patient was helped to clearly define his main problem, and how he saw professionals help in relation to this?
(4) The patient's views were challenged in order to encourage him to take greater responsibility for his condition
(5) Mr McLoughlin's plans for how he was going to spend the next week were examined in detail
(6) His risk for suicide was assessed and a referral to a psychiatrist was considered
(7) The procedure for after-hours telephone contact with the hospital was explained

Session 2
(1) The important issues for Mr McLoughlin from the previous session were reviewed
(2) Those areas in which he had been coping were identified and reinforced

(3) Discussion followed about the implications of telling his brother and others about AIDS/HIV:

- When to tell others
- Role play about how to tell them
- How he would cope if he did not tell anyone
- Whether the patient thought it would be more difficult to tell his brother now or if it would be worse if his brother found out after he died.

(4) 'Homework' task for the next session. The patient was to consider what he was to do about his medical and social management on his return to the United States

Session 3

(1) The patient was asked how he wanted to use the last session
(2) Practical issues were discussed about telling his general practitioner in the United States and linking him there with specialist medical services
(3) It was clarified which issues were now easier to manage and which still remained a problem
(4) Termination of counselling. It was put to Mr McLoughlin that there might well be further problems for him in the future. From how he had managed over the past three weeks there were indications that he would be able to cope with some issues alone. He stated that he now felt it was easier to ask for help if he could not manage

Postscript

Through the course of the sessions, the patient became less anxious, distressed and helpless, despite the fact that his health did not improve. Mr McLoughlin did not come to the hospital or contact any member of staff outside of the three sessions. The senior registrar reported that the medical examination of the patient, and talking to him, was made easier after each counselling session. The patient returned to the United States. He wrote to the senior registrar to say that he was being seen at a large AIDS Unit. He had telephoned his brother to tell him that he had AIDS and that he was homosexual. His brother travelled to the United States to see him. The patient became acutely ill a week later, and he subsequently died. On his return to the UK his brother made contact with the AIDS counsellor and an appointment was made for them to meet.

CASE I   MULTIPLE DEATHS: MAINTAINING HOPE

Description of the problem

Rupert, a 21 year old HIV antibody positive man attending a medical

outpatient clinic, became depressed and very withdrawn. He told the consultant that he had suddenly become aware of the impact on him of the deaths from AIDS of many of his friends. His brother died of AIDS four years ago. He said that this was affecting how he was managing each day.
Rupert was referred to the counsellor.

Stage of HIV infection
HIV antibody positive. Currently well

Individual's stage of life
Young adult. Single man. Openly homosexual. Living on his own
Working as an assistant in a bookshop

The individual in relation to the stage of the family's development
Parents divorced when he was 10. Both of them living in Australia
Closer to mother than to father. Brother died of AIDS four years ago
Left home and country of birth two years ago.

Principal issues to be addressed
- Other sources of social support to be identified
- What it is about the multiple deaths for this patient that is causing the greatest distress
- Use of the patient's experience of facing the deaths of his friends and his brother to explore areas where he might have gained something positive or have been inspired in any way. In addition, explore those experiences which have been negative and frightening
- If appropriate, discuss 'dreaded issues' (see Case B).

How to address these issues
The following questions were used to start a conversation in these areas and to begin to challenge Rupert's source of anxiety and depression:

(1) Who else knows you are experiencing these feelings? What is it that you are able talk to them about, and not talk about? Who else might you want to talk to? What might you see as the risk in talking to others about this? If you were not able to view these experiences in any other way, what would be the worst thing that might happen to you?
(2) Can you help me to understand what exactly it is about all of these deaths that is affecting you the most today? What is it about the experience of these deaths that has led you to feel the way you do?
(3) So, are you suggesting that from Paul's death, and the way which he faced up to it, that you have learned something? If you should have to face death, is there anything from their experiences that we can help you to avoid or to achieve?
(4) Is there anything from your own experience of these many deaths that you might be able to pass on to others that might help them?

CASE J   A MARRIAGE PROBLEM: AIDS AS THE ENTRÉ TO COUNSELLING

Description of the problem
Mrs Hart (32) telephoned an AIDS Hotline service. She asked where her husband could get an AIDS test. She said that until he was tested she would not resume a sexual relationship with him. Mrs Hart believed that her husband was having affairs with other women and that for this reason he may be "at risk" for AIDS. She wanted to know that he is "clear of AIDS".
During the brief conversation it emerged that the couple had been having marriage problems for some time

Stage of HIV infection:
Unknown as neither partner has been tested for HIV

Individual stage of life:
Adult. Mother. Given up working to care for child

The individual in relation to the stage of the family's development:
Recent marriage. Young child in family. Mrs Hart's parents both still alive

Principal issues to be addressed
- Identify the patient's main concern
- Provide information about counselling and testing sites
- Referral to a relevant professional

How the telephone interview is conducted

Client asks where she can get an AIDS test

Counsellor asks what made her want a test, and what she understands by 'the test'. Counsellor explains that the HIV antibody test in not a test for AIDS.

Client wants husband to have the test. Suspects him of having extramarital affairs. She states that she cannot speak to him as they have not spoken to one another for a few weeks.

Counsellor states that the client will have to find a way of discussing this with the husband if she wants him to have the test. The decision cannot be forced on him by anyone. The counsellor asks who else might need to be tested, such as herself or the child.

Client states she will not be tested unless her husband is tested.

Counsellor Am I right that you are worried about AIDS, but that you also have problems between you and your husband?

Client confirms that there are marriage problems.

Counsellor asks whether she would be able to talk to her general practitioner about these problems. Information about HIV testing sites and marriage guidance is given. Safer sex practices are discussed.

CASE K BEREAVEMENT: WORKING WITH SURVIVORS

Description of the problem
Mrs Murrell, aged 33, has two children aged 8 and 5, Mr Murrell died of a brain abscess six months ago. On post mortem examination he was found to be HIV antibody positive. AIDS was identified as the probable cause of his death. The first time Mrs Murrell knew about this was when she received the death certificate. Mrs Murrell has been HIV antibody negative to date. The general practitioner referred Mrs Murrell to the counsellor while he undertook to carry out the 3-monthly HIV antibody testing surveillance on her.

Stage HIV infection:
HIV antibody negative. Sexual partner of deceased HIV antibody positive man. Being retested every 3 months for 18 months in case she should seroconvert

Individual stage of life:
Young adult. Widow. Financially dependent on relatives and the State

The individual in relation to the stage of the family's development:
Single parent with 2 children
Has close contact with in-laws
Family facing up to death where there is a secret. Only she knows about her late husband's HIV antibody status

Principal issues to be addressed
- Possibility of infection with HIV for Mrs Murrell
- Identify who else has been told about Mrs Murrell's status and the possible repercussions from anyone knowing
- Consider her ideas about how her late husband might have become infected and how she is coping with this
- Help the family to face up to the father's death where there is a secret about the circumstances of his death. This is in order to prevent emotional disturbance in any member.

How to address these issues

(1) Assess what is known about the possibility of transmission of HIV to Mrs Murrell and the children. Correct misconceptions.

(2) Explore how she thinks her husband got HIV and her reactions to that now in the light of his death. If Mrs Murrell has no ideas, use hypothetical questions such as "Just say your husband had been having sexual relations with other men, would it make it easier or more difficult for you to accept his death?"

(3) Identify who else in the family knows about the cause of his death. Consider who she would like to tell and what obstacles there are in doing this. Address the advantages and disadvantages of telling others.

(4) Explore when, and how, she would consider talking to the children about the circumstances surrounding the father's death. Discuss what she now says to the children in relation to their father's death.

(5) Explore how she sees herself managing over the next two to three years. What sort of relationship does she want with her in-laws?

(6) Does she see herself as having another sexual relationship?
How does she talk to people about her husband's death?
What might she say to a future lover about her relationship with her late husband and the circumstances surrounding his death? With whom does she share her grief?

(7) Offer a further appointment for herself and the children or anyone else she wishes to bring, if this is appropriate. Offer a family therapy referral if this is indicated.

CASE L BISEXUALITY: SECRETS IN THE FAMILY

Description of the problem
An HIV antibody positive bisexual man, Mr James, consulted the AIDS counsellor as he was in a dilemma. His wife did not know that he had had male sexual partners, nor was she aware of his HIV status. Mr James would not consider using condoms when sleeping with his wife in case she became suspicious. The couple had two children.

Stage of HIV infection
HIV antibody positive and asymptomatic

Individual stage of life
Adult. Mid-life. Working

The individual in relation to the stage of the family's development
Married, and he is a parent
Has extramarital sexual relationships
Daughter preparing to leave home
Mid-life 'crisis'

Principal issues to be addressed
- Dilemma of respecting confidentiality and protecting public health
- Assess his knowledge about AIDS/HIV and transmission
- Discuss the patient's views about HIV in the context of his extramarital relationships and his relationships with his wife
- Challenge the patient's view about not informing his wife
- Discuss how he might tell his wife and implications of this for his relationship with her and with the rest of the family

How to address these issues
It helps in addressing difficult situations to ask a number of questions in order to challenge the patient's views. This may lead to his developing other ideas about how to share the information with his wife.

Question 1 What is your greatest fear in telling your wife?
If she rejected you, how do you see your future and that of your wife?
Question 2 If you decided to tell her, how do you think she might react? And how might your children react? What might be each of their greatest concerns?
Question 3 If your wife became infected with HIV how might you react? Is it worse to tell her about your infidelity, or risk her being infected and the consequences of that?
Question 4 Now that you have explained your situation to me, if you were a counsellor in my position, what would you be advising and saying to a patient?
Question 5 If your daughter was here, and you had confided in her, what do you think she would be advising you to do?
Question 6 You say that no-one else in the family knows. What makes you so sure about this?
Question 7 Have you told any of your other sexual contacts that you are married? What do you imagine they would say about the HIV risk to your wife?
Question 8 What precautions are you and your current sexual partners taking?
Question 9 If you were to decide to tell her, how would you start the conversation? Say she reacted by shouting and crying, what might you say or do?

Question 10 If your wife were to have any choice in the matter, do you think she would rather hear about your infidelity and HIV, or be kept in the dark about it and be put at risk?

Question 11 Who in the family do you think would support you the most if you were to tell them, and how would they show it?

Note
This is one approach that can be taken in an attempt to get the patient to tell his wife. If he still refuses to do so, in some circumstances, professionals may decide that public health concerns are more important than confidentiality. In circumstances such as these, the doctor might inform the wife himself.

CASE M   CULTURAL ISSUES AND HIV: AN ARRANGED MARRIAGE

Description of the problem
Mr Banjhi, a single Asian man of 23 who is HIV antibody positive, came to the haemophilia centre for treatment. He told the consultant that his parents had arranged for him to be married in six weeks. The consultant was concerned about HIV and the risk of transmission to his wife-to-be, and future children.

Stage of HIV infection:
HIV antibody positive. p24 antigen negative

Individual stage of life:
Adult. No previous sexual contacts. Working as a clerk. Living at home with his parents

The individual in relation to the family's stage of development:
Second child about to be married. Arranged marriage. Will live in parents home with wife

A framework for thinking about the principal issues
Language: Use an interpreter, where necessary. Ensure the counsellor's language and ideas are understood by the patient by checking throughout the interview. Identify the patient's words for 'intercourse', 'condoms', 'kissing' etc.
Culture: Ask the patient to describe how sex, marriage, having children and the relationship between parents and children are viewed in his particular culture.
Family: Explore the specific beliefs of the family from which the patient comes. Assess the extent to which the patient has adapted to the host culture.

Identify any potential conflicts surrounding this. Get a description of the wider kin network.

HIV in the context of a different culture: Explore what happens to people in his culture in relation to marriage and having children if there is any known disability. Consider what is told to the future parents-in-law or wife about a disability.

Specific dilemmas: Help the patient to consider the risks of unprotected intercourse and the possible consequences of revealing HIV after the wedding. Encourage him to bring his future spouse to a further session. Emphasize the HIV risk to sexual partners and future children. Check what the patient knows in stages. Provide opportunities for further discussion. Provide a link, without breaching confidentiality, with other people in a similar situation. The counsellor should consult with, or refer patient to, a colleague who shares the same cultural background as the patient. Discuss with the patient whom they would like to counsel them. Some people from whatever background will, for example, insist on being seen only by a doctor.

CASE N   ADOLESCENT AT RISK: FAMILY CONCERNS

Description of the problem
The parents of a 15 year old girl have been referred to the counsellor by the general practitioner as they are worried about their daughter's behaviour. She is mixing with a crowd who may be using intravenous drugs. They also suspect that she is having sexual intercourse with several young men. The couple also have a 14 year old boy.

Stage of HIV infection
At risk. Not tested

Individual stage of life
Adolescent. Leaving school. Sexually active. Ambivalent about being an adult or a child

The individual in relation to the family's stage of development
Parents in mid-life. Adolescent children at home
Both parents were themselves only children in their own families
Parents reaching the stage where they are caring for their parents as well as their children

Principal issues to be addressed

- Identify the main concern of each parent
- Ask what has been done about the problems so far and with what effect

- Enquire as to how the parents might manage if their child did have HIV
- Find out how the parents have dealt with issues about birth control, sex, relationships and AIDS/HIV, with each of their children
- Identify who else, apart from the general practitioner, is aware of their concern (for example, teacher, school nurse)
- Develop a strategy for bringing in both children for a family session with the parents

How to address these issues

The following questions may be used to address some of these issues:

(1) Of all of the problems you have told us about today, which concerns you the most? Do your views differ from those of your wife, about this concern? If your children were here, what would be each of their main concerns? Who else is aware of these concerns? What would help you most in solving this problem? Which of the two of you is most concerned?

(2) Have you spoken to your daughter about your worry? How did she react? Have you spoken to anyone else about these issues? What would each of your own parent's view be of the problem, and how do you think each of them would suggest you handle this?

(3) What do you know about AIDS and HIV? Who in the family do you think would be the most affected by AIDS? In what way? What is your greatest fear for yourselves? What is your greatest fear for your family? How do each of you see yourself managing these fears?

(4) Which of the two of you takes the main responsibility for talking about sex and relationships with your children? Who else do you think your children talk to? Where else might they get their information? Is AIDS ever spoken about at home?

(5) Would you be able to talk to anyone in the school about the drug and sex problem? If AIDS/HIV were not an added problem, who would you turn to about your concern about drugs?

(6) If your daughter knew that you were coming here today, what do you think she would imagine we would be discussing? How might she react if she knew you were here? Does your son know that you have worries about your daughter? Do you think your son might be at any risk for HIV? Who, of all the family and your own parents, has the most influence on your daughter? What would they be advising you to do?

(7) Do you think you are more likely to solve this problem by discussing it with the children or without them? How do you think you might persuade your daughter to come here to see us? Which of the two of you might have the greatest chance of achieving this with her? Are you more afraid of losing her if she runs away from home and gets caught up further in this business, or having a huge confrontation with her?

(8) We would like you to come with the whole family because in this way we can get the most information, and this helps us to develop more ideas about how to help you.

CASE O   FEAR OF AIDS: WORRIED, BUT WELL

Description of the problem
Miss Lindsey (24) was referred by her general practitioner to the counsellor. She had complained to him several times in the past that he was not taking her fear of infection with the AIDS virus seriously. In spite of his careful questioning about Miss Lindsey's past personal, sexual, medical, and drug history, the general practitioner was unable to reassure her that he could find no reason to believe that she could possibly have been infected in the past. Miss Lindsey admitted to having worries about many aspects of her health.

Stage of HIV Infection
Worried about AIDS. Has not been tested

Individual stage of life
Single. Young adult. Living at home. Dress designer
No previous sexual relationships
At age 14 was anorexic for 2 years

The individual in relation to the stage of the family's development
Parents elderly in late mid-life. Only child. No other siblings. Daughter still living at home. Close relationship with father

Principal issues to be addressed

- Review current knowledge about AIDS/HIV and need for information
- Assess which activities that might have put her at risk
- Review of past individual and family histories
- Explore the consequences of a positive or negative HIV antibody test result
- Come to some understanding as to why she has come now (for example, influence of media campaign, friend has AIDS)
- Offer HIV antibody test if appropriate. (See Pre-and post-test counselling interview, Chapter 7)

How to address these issues

Session One
1. Ask the patient what concern it is that has brought her to the clinic.

2. Identify what she believes has put her at risk for HIV. Detailed discussion about sex and drug activities, and past medical history.

3. Ask the patient what she knows about AIDS: give information.

4. Ask patient what she knows about the HIV antibody test.

5. Discuss the implications of the HIV antibody test.

6. Ask if she would be reassured if the result was negative
Discuss how she might cope if it was positive.

7. Offer a further appointment. Patient told to decide whether she
wants the HIV antibody test in the interim.

Session Two

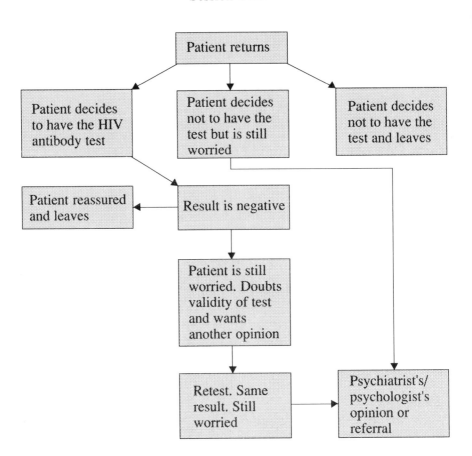

CASE P   FORMING RELATIONSHIPS IN THE CONTEXT OF AIDS/HIV

Description of the problem
Brad, 21, made an appointment to see the AIDS counsellor on the advice of a friend. He said he wanted a chance to talk to someone about AIDS-related worries. In the first interview Brad said that although he did not feel he was at risk for AIDS/HIV, his worries about becoming infected had prevented him from pursuing the type of social life that might have led to his forming relationships.

Stage of HIV infection:
Presumed HIV antibody negative. Not tested

Individual stage of life:
Young adult left home. Starting a career. Recently left university

The individual in relation to the family's stage of development:
Brad and his older brother live away from home
Younger sister still lives with the parents

Principal issues to be addressed

- Provide an opportunity to talk about his concerns
- Help Brad to identify, amongst these problems, which is the most important and pressing
- Get Brad to define quite specifically what he wants to achieve through the counselling session
- Assess how the fear of AIDS has affected his ability to form and maintain relationships
- Offer a view that this may be a common problem for many people of his age and in his circumstances
- The counsellor must be ever-alert to the possibility that long-term counselling might be a substitute for these relationships he is not able to develop elsewhere. This may be prevented if the focus of the counselling is clear; if a structure is provided; time boundaries are set; and the contract is not open-ended

How to address some of the issues
The following are some questions which may be used by the counsellor to be begin to talk about the above concerns:
(1) What is it that you most want to discuss today?
What is it that prompted you to come now?
What do you think your friend had in mind for you in coming here today?
(2) Of these problems you have mentioned which is the most difficult for you to handle?

If you didn't face this problem now, what else might be going on in your life, and what else might be worrying you?

What would your parents guess is your main concern at the moment?
What would their view be of your problem?

Do you think that your brother and sister might have similar concerns given that they might also be at risk for AIDS?

(3) What are you hoping for today from this session?

How will you know when you have been helped?

What will have happened for us all to feel that we no longer need to meet?

(4) Tell me what the main difficulty is for you being gay and 21?

How does you fear of AIDS affect this?

Do you think there could possibly be any benefits from peoples' worries about AIDS?

Do you think that the worry about AIDS and sex may make people have to talk more to one another? And how do you see this affecting peoples' ability to have long-term relationships?

If AIDS wasn't about do you think you would have the same difficulties in meeting others and forming relationships?

Do you think that other people may have the same difficulties as you?

If you were to enter into a relationship and there was the possibility of it becoming sexual, would you be able to talk about safer sex practices?

(5) If, for example, you were not able to have the sort of relationship you are talking about, how do you see yourself using your time over the next year or two? What qualities do you think someone else would look for in you if they were interested in forming a relationship with you?

CASE Q   MAINTAINING HOPE IN THE FACE OF LIFE-THREATENING ILLNESS

What is maintaining hope?

It is implicit in any caring relationship that support and encouragement will be provided to the patient, the family, and close friends. There is seldom 100 per cent certainty about the course and outcome of any illness. Even with a condition like AIDS there is the possibility that new treatments will become available in the lifetime of any patient. The meaning which the patient attaches to a message of encouragement depends on who is giving it. When a member of the health care team encourages a patient this is also a communication to the patient that there may be scientific advances from which he might benefit. For this reason the message carries special authority.

The following are examples of what is sometimes conveyed to patients:

- The patient should be a 'winner' and not a 'loser'
- The patient should always look cheerful
- They should keep fighting in the face of all adversity
- They should 'pull up their socks'
- New drugs and treatments may become available. 'There is always hope on the horizon'
- 'Be positive'
- 'You are better off than that chap over there'

The impact of these messages on patients:
Much has got to do with *when* a message of hope is given to a patient. If the message is given when someone feels depressed and hopeless the effect may be to stop them talking about their fears, worries and feelings. This in turn can increase the patient's feelings of isolation and anxiety.

Ways of addressing situations that may seem hopeless and serious
Although words of encouragement are sometimes appropriate there are other ways in which to respond to and comfort patients who are distressed:
(1) Sit and listen to whatever is said, no matter how compelling it might be to respond by giving reassurance.
(2) Gestures, such as:

- Where you sit in relation to the patient (on a chair or at the end of the bed)
- Physical contact such as touch, at appropriate moments
- Talking about their greatest fears rather than finding some reason to leave the room at that moment.

(3) Convey hope by giving a considered message to the patient at the end of the session. The message should include a summary of:

- The counsellor's view of how the patient is managing
- The patient's concerns
- The themes that have emerged during the session
- Some of the behaviour seen during the session
- Some important statements made by the patient
- The 'normality' of the patient's response should be emphasized
- The counsellor should always find at least one positive comment to make about how the patient has been managing. It means more to the patient if this statement relates to what has been seen and heard in the session. One might say: "Even though you have been so unwell lately, you have still prepared your own meals. That reflects your ability to stay independant as long as possible. In the past you have said how important that is for you"

- The message at the end of the session conveys to patients that their ideas and concerns have been heard and considered.

This summary can give a new perspective to the patient.

Example
The following is an example of a summary message that might be given.
"Paul, from what I have heard from you today it sounds to me that you have had to face many difficulties in the last month. You said to me that you are worried about your illness, and this in turn makes you feel very depressed, hopeless and unable to make decisions. In my experience of working with people who face life-threatening illness one would be surprised if they did not react in a way similar to the way you have. It seems you have the expectation of yourself that you always have to be cheerful and to be seen to be coping. I am not sure where this view comes from. Perhaps we can discuss this in another session.

From what you have told me, during the last two weeks, you have managed to get to two parties. On another occasion you decided to cancel your arrangement and rather to stay at home and listen to records instead. Even though you say you are depressed and that you cannot make decisions, it seems to me that on these occasions you have been quite able to decide what is best for you at that time, even if it has meant being on your own.

At the beginning of the session you told me how hopeless you feel. I'm very impressed that you have been able to do all that you have done, and found some enjoyment despite your feeling so hopeless".

CASE R   ENGAGING OTHER MEMBERS OF THE FAMILY IN COUNSELLING SESSIONS

Description of the problem
Barry, 21, was found to be HIV antibody positive five months ago. He has recently recovered from an episode of *Pneumocystis carinii* pneumonia, and so a diagnosis of AIDS had been confirmed. While he was an inpatient the main focus of his conversations with the counsellor was how he could resume contact with his family and tell them about his diagnosis. This would also mean talking more openly about his being gay.

Stage of HIV infection:
AIDS diagnosis recently confirmed

Individual's stage in life:
Young adult. No permanent relationships. Starting a career as a lawyer

The individual in relation to the stage of the family's development:
Left home. Older sister married. Younger sister working as a secretary
Both living away from home
Parents looking after ailing maternal grandmother

Principal issues to be addressed
- Assess the patient's view of his relationship with his family
- Explore how he would like the relationship to be with the members of his family
- Consider how the patient can get closer to his family

How to address these issues
(1) How do members of your family usually respond when someone is ill?
(2) When you have been ill in the past what did they do?
(3) How do you see your relationship with your mother (father, sister or grandmother)?
(4) Is this any different to how you would have described it six months ago?
(5) Would your mother agree with this view?
(6) How might your father describe the relationship between you and your mother?
(7) If both of your sisters were here today, and they heard these views, what might each want to say about this?
(8) What is your grandmother's view of your relationship with your parents?
(9) If you were able to choose, how would you like the relationship to be between you and your mother (father, sisters, grandmother)?
(10) Who else knows that you are in hospital?
(11) Who else knows you have AIDS?
(12) What might their views be if they knew?
(13) What has prevented your telling them so far?
(14) What in your view is the main obstacle which prevents this?
(15) If things were to be different between you and your father how would this help you?
(16) What would you most want now from each member of your family?
(17) Do you think that having more contact with your parents would make them more or less concerned about you?
(18) How would they show this, and how might this affect you?
(19) When might it be preferable to start talking to them about these issues?
(20) Now, whilst you are well, or if you were perhaps to become ill again?
(21) If you were to begin to talk to someone in your family about AIDS, who would you choose first?
(22) What is it that makes it easier to talk to your younger sister rather than your older sister?
(23) What do you most fear will happen if you talk to them about AIDS?
(24) Who do you think will take the news best and in what way?
(25) What might be your parents' greatest concern when they hear you have AIDS?

(26) What might help them most with this?

(27) If your parents were to react by rejecting you what would help you to cope with this?

(28) Who else might you turn to for comfort and support if things did not work out with the family?

(29) How could you best maintain the relationship with your parents in such a way that you had contact with them but did not feel overwhelmed?

(30) If it were not AIDS, but another life-threatening illness, would it make it easier to make contact with your family? In what way?

Postscript

Three weeks after this interview Barry telephoned his mother to tell her he had been ill, but he did not say he had AIDS. He subsequently visited the family. His father asked him directly if he had AIDS. Barry reported that it was easier to say 'yes' than he had previously imagined it would be. His parents, although very distressed, have tried to support him. The discussion now is whether, when and how to tell his sisters. He has arranged to come and see the counsellor with his parents.

Although there were no answers to many of the questions, hearing them helped Barry to think about many issues in the family. This prepared him to handle the situation with more confidence.

CASE S   COUNSULTATION TO EXPERT COUNSELLORS: AIDS COUNSELLING CONSULTATION TO A PSYCHIATRIC TEAM

Description of the problem

The registrar in a psychiatric hospital telephoned the AIDS Counselling Unit asking for advice about testing a patient for HIV. The registrar felt that the patient, a young man of 22, was at considerable risk. Not only had he used intravenous drugs and shared needles in the past, but the patient also had a history of manic-depressive illness. There were times when he had been very promiscuous while he was in a manic phase. The registrar felt that he had to exclude HIV as a possible cause of his present psychotic episode, but that he was not sure about how to begin to discuss this with the patient.

Principal issues to be addressed

The psychiatric team

- Identify areas of major concern to the team in relation to this patient (for example, the risk of infection of other patients and staff)

- Enquire as to whether the patient would be able to engage in full and meaningful discussion about issues, and whether each of them believes that the patient would be able to cope with a positive HIV antibody test result. Identify who else in the patient's family needs to be involved in making any decisions
- Consider how to enable members of the psychiatric team to do what they are best trained to do; that is, talk to their patient, and incorporate all the AIDS issues into their meetings with the patient

The patient

- There is a need for discussion about AIDS/HIV transmission and prevention
- Identify who else may be at risk if the patient were HIV antibody positive
- Assess how the patient might cope if he were HIV antibody positive and what actions he might be able to take to prevent other people being infected by him
- Identify who else is most able to influence the patient (family, friends, psychiatric team).

Outcome
The counsellor met the psychiatric team (consultant, registrar, psychiatric nurse and social worker). It was decided that the patient would be seen by the registrar with the counsellor present. The patient was not psychotic at the time. The registrar conducted the interview with the patient and referred to the counsellor whenever he was not sure about a point. In this way the registrar learned more about AIDS issues and the counsellor learned something about this type of psychiatric patient. An HIV antibody test was done with the patient's consent and the result was negative. It was decided that there should be further test in three months time as the patient had had sexual intercourse with three different people the previous week.

CASE T   HIV ANTIBODY TESTING IN ANTENATAL CLINICS

Reasons for offering antibody testing in antenatal clinics
In order to monitor heterosexual transmission of AIDS, and in the wake of the heterosexual AIDS epidemic, especially in Africa, it is inevitable that HIV antibody testing will be carried out in antenatal clinics. There are two procedures for this. The first is through anonymous screening, and the second is through informed consent. Irrespective of the approach taken, staff in antenatal clinics will have to consider many of the issues that are described in this case.

There are specific reasons as to why the HIV antibody test should be offered to mothers who are pregnant, and perhaps to the father:

1. Transmission of HIV must be prevented. In the context of antenatal clinics this is with regard to transmission from:
   - mother to unborn child
   - one sexual partner to another
   - health care staff who come into contact with patients' blood, and where invasive procedures have to be performed.
2. Although there is no conclusive evidence, there are reports that for an asymptomatic HIV antibody positive mother, pregnancy itself may increase her chances of developing an AIDS-related illness or AIDS.
3. Epidemiological data is essential for monitoring the spread of HIV to all groups, including the heterosexual population and to children, in order that preventative strategies can be developed and provision be made for the care of infected parents and their children.
4. Decisions will need to be made as to whether or not an infected mother ought to proceed with the pregnancy.
5. The obstetric staff need to be aware of possible risks of infection at delivery and to decide on the level of protection needed.
6. Discussion will have to follow as to whether or not the sexual partner/father will be informed and encouraged to be tested.
7. Follow-up care and surveillance for a known HIV antibody positive mother and her family will need to be provided.
8. The extent that an obstetrician and midwife are prepared to sanction natural childbirth will need to be considered.

Specific issues in HIV antibody testing in antenatal clinics

Infection control
Staff working with expectant mothers must be reassured first about their occupational risk. As in all other areas of medical care, infection control procedures must be referred to.

Busy clinics
Counselling in relation to HIV in antenatal clinics will increase the workload of the staff. Specialist counsellors can be called upon, but staff in these clinics will need to develop an introductory counselling repertoire suitable for these clinics. An example will be given later in this case.

Timing of the HIV antibody test
Ideally, HIV antibody testing should be carried out before pregnancy, through liaison with general practitioners and family planning clinics. HIV antibody testing can also be carried out on pregnant women. This should be done as early on in pregnancy as possible so consideration can be given to termination of the pregnancy should the need arise. This may mean booking women into antenatal clinics at an earlier stage than is usually the practice.

It must always be remembered that, because of the 'window period' of incubation time for developing HIV antibodies, women may need need to be retested throughout the course of the pregnancy if the exposure has been very recent.

There are fewer options for the mother and also for the obstetrician if HIV antibody testing is performed at a late stage in pregnancy.

Management of the HIV antibody positive mother

Views about termination of pregnancy must be explored. 'Dreaded issues' need to be raised with mothers who decide to continue with the pregnancy, as described in Chapter 7 and in Case A in this chapter.

The need to use precautions during sexual intercourse must be emphasized during the course of pregnancy. Consideration must be given as to whether the father will be informed and tested.

A physician would need to monitor the mother from an HIV point of view and a paediatrician should be introduced to the mother at an early stage.

From the counselling point of view all efforts should be made to enable the mother to make informed decisions.

Management of the HIV antibody positive father

If the mother is known to be HIV antibody positive there is a chance that the father will also be HIV antibody positive. The obstetrician would have to discuss with the mother the need to test the father for HIV.

Special consideration needs to be given to cases where the father is known to be HIV antibody positive and the mother is negative. Seroconversion of the mother may take place during the course of pregnancy which also has implications for the fetus. In such cases the mother should be repeatedly tested throughout pregnancy and also for a period thereafter.

What to include in counselling and examples of leading questions
(see also Chapter 8 and Chapter 9 case A, for more extensive discussion about pre- and post-test counselling).

A. *Introduction to HIV antibody testing.*
"Mrs Thompson, as you know in our clinic we offer the HIV antibody test as a routine to all expectant mothers. What do you understand about why we offer this test?"

B. *Knowledge about AIDS and transmission of HIV*
"How might someone in your position come to be infected with HIV?"
"What do you know about AIDS?"
"What do you understand about the risk to the unborn child
if the mother has HIV?"
"If the father is positive what do you know about the risk to the mother and the unborn child?"

C. *Knowledge about HIV antibody test*
"What do you know about the HIV antibody test?"
(see Chapters 7, 8 and 9)

D. *Assessing the risk for HIV*
Explore issues relating to past sexual practices, drug use, blood transfusion and artificial insemination by donor (AID). Assess whether there has been rape or sexual abuse in the past.
"Have you had any sexual contacts outside of this relationship in the past?"
"Do you think your husband or partner has been at risk in any way?"

E. *Talking about having the HIV antibody test*
"Do you agree to have the test?"
"You say that you do not want to have the test. What do you fear most about having the test?"
"Given, you are not prepared to have the test we are going to treat you as if you are HIV antibody positive from an infection control point of view. What are your views about this?"
"If your partner were here today would he agree with your decision not to have the test?"
"If your result were positive what would your views be about terminating the pregnancy? Would your partner agree with this?"
"If the result were negative, and you knew there might be some risk, would you agree to have another test in three months time?"
"When we give you the result would you like to come on your own or with your partner?"

CASE U   A GROUP FOR HIV ANTIBODY POSITIVE PATIENTS: CONVENING, LEADING AND LEARNING

The background
The idea of a group for patients who have HIV came from several patients who were attending a clinic. They wanted to meet with other people who were in a similar position to themselves to hear how the others were managing. The counsellor agreed to convene and lead the group. Twelve patients came to the first meeting and have continued to meet every three months.

Issues to be addressed

- Decision about leadership
- The task and purpose of the group
- Confidentiality

- Frequency of meetings
- Structure of sessions
- Venue
- Time of day
- Length of sessions

Procedure for a structured group

A. Group leader describes the rules of the group:
    (1) Only one person talks at a time
    (2) Each member takes responsibility for what he or she says
    (3) What is known about the individual's medical and social situation is confidential and is not discussed by the leader/counsellor. Strict confidentiality is to be observed
    (4) Anything that is discussed in the group should be regarded as confidential to the group and should not be discussed outside
                        (5 minutes)

B. The group leader introduces himself and asks each person to say:
    (1) Who they are
    (2) What is the main reason that brought them to the group
                        (10 minutes)

C. Each person states what they would most want to discuss that evening. The ideas are written up on a board
                        (5 minutes)

D. Divide into three groups. Each group chooses 2 topics from the board to discuss. One person is nominated to take notes. The sub-groups are given the task of:
    (1) Discussing the issues
    (2) Considering what has helped them to manage that particular situation and what they feel remains a difficulty for them
                        (40 minutes)

E. The large group reconvenes. The notekeeeper from each group reports the points that emerged from discussion in the small group
                        (10 minutes)

F. Open forum for discussion. The leader ensures that everyone is able to participate
                        (15 minutes)

G. Ideas are solicited for the next meeting
                        (5 minutes)

H. Each member states:
   (1) What suprised him or her the most from the evening's discussion
   (2) What has been most helpful
   (3) What remains a problem

(20 minutes)

I. The group leader summarizes the main themes of the session. He reinforces any initiatives that people are taking themselves. A date and time for next meeting is set.

(5 minutes)

CASE V   GROUPS FOR PROFESSIONALS: STAFF SUPPORT

Description of the problem

All groups of workers may benefit from setting aside time to discuss professional issues. In the field of AIDS/HIV this can have particular relevance. This is because:

(1) It is a new field and there may be uncertainty amongst staff about how to deal with the many and ever-evolving issues
(2) Many of these people may have not worked together previously
(3) The work itself may be stressful because:

   • Resources may be in short supply
   • Some members of staff may fear being infected
   • Many of the people who have AIDS are young

One procedure for running staff groups (See also Chapter 11)
(1) Meetings should be held regularly
(2) For optimal benefit the meetings should be attended by all members of the team or unit
(3) The head of department must give his or her authority for such meetings otherwise the objectives of the group are unlikely to be achieved
(4) Meetings should provide an opportunity for discussing some of the following:

   • How each person is carrying out his task
   • What each person's main concern is in relation to the work with patients
   • What each person's main concern is in relation to colleagues (for-example, overlapping roles)

- Identifying those problems staff may have in dealing with patients, their family and contacts
- Reviewing a case after a patient has died
- Future projects, such as an introduction of a new drug, loss of inpatient beds, or a new government publicity campaign
- Considering the unit's relationship with other agencies and departments

Principles
(1) The focus in these sessions should always relate to problems arising from the work situation. It is inappropriate to concentrate on personal issues.
(2) It is not sufficient to just identify problems. The group leader must ensure that ideas and strategies are discussed for overcoming problems.

10
Setting up a clinically based
AIDS counselling service

There may be difficulties in setting up any new service in an existing organisation. AIDS is a complex medical problem that places a strain on existing resources and demands co-ordinated specialist services. AIDS Counselling Units have been introduced into some hospitals. Experience gained from the setting up of one such counselling service may be of value to those contemplating the same or thinking about introducing other new services into a hospital.

Assessing Needs
Services are usually only provided according to identified needs. An assessment of needs in relation to AIDS/HIV is best made by considering some of the following:

Existing demands for services need to be assesed in all units of the hospital and the wider district.
Current epidemiology The Department of Health and Social Security, and the Centre for Disease Surveillance and Control regularly circulate figures to health authorities of known AIDS/HIV cases in any region. Known risk factors are also reported.
Projected epidemiological trends Such trends may help in planning. The decision as to whether a special 'AIDS ward' should be designated, may be based on this.
Local problems Some districts may have special needs. In some areas there may be a large regional haemophilia centre, or in another there may be a busy sexually transmitted diseases clinic. Apart from providing services for those found to be HIV antibody positive, the size of the 'worried well' population should always be considered. There may, for example, be a large number of young people living in the area. As the decision to offer the HIV antibody test becomes more routine, so demand for counselling expertise will increase.

Problems inherent in establishing a new service
Practical, managerial and relationship difficulties often accompany the development of any new service. AIDS counselling services present challenges in some of the following areas:

Staffing
Managers may have to decide what the best professional background should be for a counsellor. Nurses, psychologists, social workers, doctors and others

are in AIDS counselling posts in different districts. The final choice of the managers may be influenced by financial constraints; the suitablity of existing personnel; or a belief that a certain profession is best suited to the task.

Management and accountability
There is, at present, no professional structure for AIDS counsellors. Decisions will need to be made about clinical and managerial accountability according to the professional background of the postholder.

Physical location
Many AIDS counsellors work in sexually transmitted diseases clinics which have an outpatient remit. As an increasing number of medical specialities contribute to the care of these patients, a sexually transmitted diseases clinic may not, in the future, be the optimum location for an AIDS counsellor. In coming years, counsellors will increasingly have to make stronger links with all hospital departments. There may be some advantage for counselling services to be accommodated separately from any existing department.

Evaluation
Any service needs to be evaluated. Managers should negotiate with counsellors about the task and objectives of the service, and how these can best be assessed. It is much easier to evaluate patient care where the outcome is 'recovery', 'chronic illness' or 'death'. AIDS counselling is less easily evaluated. Some variables might be 'improved patient management', 'better quality of life', 'less psychiatric morbidity in survivors and family members', or 'decreased incidence of HIV in the community'.

Envy
While most health authorities are having to manage cuts in budgets, AIDS may be seen by many to be a field where resources are in abundance. Counsellors and their managers need to address the impact of the new service on the existing environment. Relationships with other members of staff in different units could become strained. Envy may also surface in the form of professional rivalry. Nurses and social workers, for example, might view counselling as being their traditional remit.

Rejection
There might be some members of staff who do not have a special interest in AIDS/HIV. They may have a particular view about homosexuals or drug abusers, or they may have other specialist interests. It is important that managers first survey the needs and views of staff in order to identify potential problem areas which might later interfere with the relationship between the counsellor and different units. Concurrence over the objectives, role and operation of counselling service will need to be established in order that inappropriate referrals are not made and unreasonable expectations of the counsellor do not arise.

Interviewing existing staff

The views and needs of key members of different departments should be surveyed in relation to a new AIDS counselling service. This can help focus on some of the specific and unique problems outlined above. There is the potential to reduce interpersonal problems stemming from a lack of concurrence over the function, activities and task of the new service. The aims of the discussion between managers and heads of departments are to:

- Assess the specific needs of each consultant and head of department in relation to AIDS counselling
- Elicit their ideas of AIDS counselling and how this could fit into the work of their department
- Gather some information about how referrals would be made and by whom
- Identify who else in each unit has experience working with AIDS/HIV patients, and who has specific skills in relation to counselling and bereavement issues, so as not to duplicate existing resources
- Outline how case notes would be kept and confidentiality preserved.
- Decide how feedback and evaluation of counselling meetings would be undertaken
- Correct erroneous views about AIDS counselling in relation to this unique health problem

The following is a series of questions that may be put to different senior members of staff in order to achieve some of these aims.

Questions about the need for counselling

1. Do you have need of a counsellor?
2. Can you think of a situation where you might need a counsellor?
3. Who else on your staff might agree with this? Who might disagree?
4. What is unique about the needs of patients under your care? What would be important for us to know in relation to the AIDS/HIV problems you face in your work setting?
5. What statistics would you want the AIDS counsellor to keep in relation to your patient?

Questions to help explore the scope of counselling

1. What might you expect of an AIDS counsellor in relation to your patients?
2. How might AIDS counselling help in the management of your patients? In what way might it interfere with this?
3. What problems might you expect with patients? What would you expect of an AIDS counsellor in relation to these?
4. Who else might benefit by referring patients to the AIDS counsellor?
5. Are there specific issues that you would prefer AIDS counsellors not to discuss with patients?
6. What do you think is the single most important contribution an AIDS counsellor could make to your patients? And their family? And your staff?

7. How might you deal with some of the problems of these patients if there was no counselling service?

8. How have similar problems been dealt with on your ward in the past? Which staff have appropriate experience?

9. What issues for patients do you think fall outside the scope of both the medical and the AIDS counselling service?

Questions to help think about the referral procedure

1. When making the referral, what information do you think would be the most important for the AIDS counsellor to know?

2. At which point in time do you think a patient would need to see an AIDS counsellor? What would indicate to you that a referral to an AIDS counsellor might be appropriate?

3. What clues do you think a patient would give you to indicate they had a problem?

4. What would convince you that a patient did not need AIDS counselling?

5. At what point in their illness do you think a patient should first see a counsellor? At what point might they be least suited for this?

Questions about feedback from and evaluation of sessions

1. How might you know if the patient was benefiting from AIDS counselling? What clues would you look for?

2. How can the issue of confidentiality with the patient be dealt with in relation to giving you some feedback about the sessions?

3. What information would be most useful to you in relation to counselling sessions?

4. How often would you want feedback about counselling sessions?

5. What would you like the counsellor to achieve for you to think that the case can be closed? What behaviour from the patient would indicate this?

Questions addressing the relationships between the counsellor and other members of staff on the ward

1. How would you see your staff working with the AIDS counsellor?

2. Which of your colleagues would agree most strongly with your views about this? Who the least?

3. Who else on your staff counsels these patients?

4. Who else on your staff is keen to work with these patients? Who the least?

5. Who on your staff might be interested in sitting in on sessions with the counsellor in order to learn more about counselling?

Questions relating counselling to the wider system

1. Do you see a place for staff counselling in relation to the AIDS/HIV problem?

2. Who on your staff might be able to take over from the AIDS counsellor? To whom would members of your staff go if they encountered difficulties arising from counselling?

3. At what point might others, such as the family or lovers, be involved in counselling?

4. What has helped your staff so far to deal with the problem of AIDS? If the counsellor were to note that the patient was receiving conflicting messages from members of staff, how might you want them to deal with this?

11
Managing staff stress in a clinical setting

The impact on health care staff of having to work with patients with AIDS/HIV is, in some cases, considerable. This in turn affects the morale and efficiency of any team. In the first five years of the AIDS problem, much of the stress resulting from this work stemmed from the fact that AIDS was a new clinical problem. Sexually transmitted diseases clinics were not essentially designed for inpatient care nor for dealing with a growing number of young and seriously ill patients.

The sources of stress are now usually quite specific and identifiable. In this short chapter the ways in which stress is manifest are identified and some strategies are outlined for dealing with work-related stress.

Current sources of stress

Unanticipated and stressful tasks

For example:
1. Talking to patients about life-threatening illnesses
2. Taking a sex history
3. Caring for a large number of acutely ill people whose condition may lead to death
4. Having to help young people face disfigurement, disability and death
5. Having to give information that is incomplete, or may later prove to be incorrect because of the rapidly increasing knowledge about AIDS and HIV
6. Not being able to reassure patients about their condition
7. Not having adequate or sufficient skills for counselling patients, their relatives and friends

Management and organizational difficulties

For example:
1. Pressure at work from insufficient and inadequate resources, such as counselling rooms, telephones and secretarial help
2. Not being consulted by managers when policy decisions are being made
3. Unclear or poorly defined work boundaries between members of staff
4. Pressure at work to either do more research or more clinical work
5. Pressure at work to give lectures and lead seminars
6. The lack of suitable supervisors or people with whom one can discuss work issues in this rapidly growing field

Personal and home issues that intrude into the work situation

For example:
1. Anxiety about being infected with HIV by patients in the clinical setting
2. Anxiety of the spouse, lover or close friends of the professional about being infected and the social stigma that is associated with AIDS
3. Over-identification of health-care staff with patients; many professionals are themselves young, sexually active and at some personal risk from being infected with HIV
4. Difficulty in achieving a balance between time spent at home and at work

How work-related stress is manifested

Work-related stress becomes evident in both the home and workplace of professionals. Some members of staff pose a dilemma about whether or not to talk about work-related issues at home with their family, lover or friends. At times, this source of support might be unavailable because either the family and others do not want to hear any more about AIDS or the professional is anxious about sharing problems because they fear this will burden or alienate these people from them. In addition, these professionals often report having less time and energy for their friends and social activities.

In the workplace, some professionals complain of 'burnout'. General inefficiency becomes evident; staff come late for meetings; there is increased absenteeism and morale is generally low. Emotionally, some members of staff feel more 'brittle' and they become short-tempered; they are less capable of doing their job effectively and efficiently. Some are unable to make decisions about which tasks and responsibilities require urgent attention and which can be delegated to colleagues. 'Burnout' is seen to arise when there is a discrepancy between the demands of the job and the ability of a member of staff to fulfil the demands for a variety of possible reasons. If this imbalance is not redressed, morale is affected; a high turnover of staff may follow and tasks are not adequately executed.

How to manage staff stress in a clinical setting (see Case V, Chapter 9)

Many professionals in the AIDS field have reported that one solution to managing staff stress is to organize regular meetings for all members of staff, at all levels, in order to express their concerns. If this is done decisions must be made about:

1. **The composition of the group**: should it be all medical consultants or should there be, for example, a mix of professionals and others, such as receptionists and secretaries?
2. **The frequency of the meetings**: should these be monthly or every three months?
3. **The leadership of the group**: will it be different facilitators from within the unit, an outside facilitator, or the head of the unit?

4. **The purpose and task of the group**: is it, for example, to discuss practical matters only or is there likely to be an opportunity for personal issues to be raised?

Whatever the form of these meetings there are several guidelines that should be adhered to in order to increase the likelihood of the meeting being successful and useful. First, the head of the unit should be advised about the meetings and he or she should sanction them. It is preferable if he attends. Second, a focus should be kept. The group should endeavour to solve problems and find solutions to whatever issue is raised, and avoid blaming or making personal attacks on colleagues. Third, the impact of any decisions or new ideas of other professionals and departments with which one works should always be considered. Often solutions to problems in units are the start of a bigger problem in the institution. A decision to create an 'AIDS Ward', for example, may be against the interests of colleagues in other fields who are trying to economize and make substantial cuts in other departments.

Opportunities should always be provided for individual members of staff to approach a head of department with specific concerns. The Occupational Health Unit of the hospital can also be used by staff if they have AIDS or work-related worries. It should be noted that a few members of staff complain about being overwhelmed by grief when a patient dies, and invariably, it is those members of staff who have formed personal relationships with patients where this most often happens. This is to be expected where patients and staff are young and when patients are well-known to the unit. Appropriate ways should be found for members of staff to share their own grief. They may need to share it with the survivors of the patient, a staff counsellor, or someone outside of the clinical setting.

In Conclusion

AIDS counselling, and indeed the whole task of caring for patients with AIDS/HIV and their family, lovers and friends, depends on multidisciplinary teamwork. The single most important resource of any AIDS unit is its staff. Good morale among members of staff often leads to exemplary standards of care and treatment for patients. The complex nature of AIDS work has resulted in large numbers of professionals having to come together to contribute to patients' care. This is, in effect, a large scale experiment in interdisciplinary liaison in the general hospital and in the community. Many new ideas highlighted by AIDS/HIV will help to advance clinical practice in other fields.

What is known about AIDS/HIV will continue to evolve and change. Approaches to counselling patients with AIDS/HIV will have to be adapted as the natural history of HIV infection unfolds. Like in most areas of medicine, there can never be 100 per cent certainty about so many issues. The approach outlined in this book is of specific use in helping patients to live with uncertainty. The ideas put forward may have application in counselling patients who have other medical conditions where uncertainty prevails.

Index